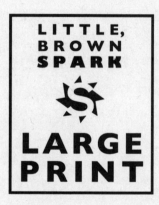

LITTLE,
BROWN
SPARK

LARGE
PRINT

ALSO BY DR. JOSH AXE

Keto Diet Cookbook

Keto Diet

Eat Dirt

THE
COLLAGEN
DIET

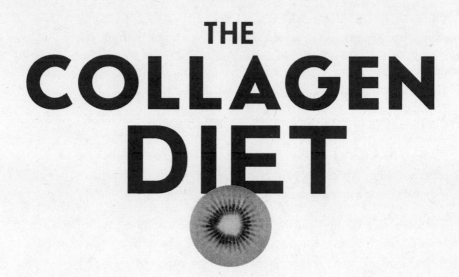

A 28-Day Plan for Sustained Weight Loss,
Glowing Skin, Great Gut Health,
and a Younger You

DR. JOSH AXE

LITTLE, BROWN SPARK
LARGE PRINT EDITION

Copyright © 2019 by Dr. Josh Axe

Hachette Book Group supports the right to free expression and the value of copyright. The purpose of copyright is to encourage writers and artists to produce the creative works that enrich our culture.

The scanning, uploading, and distribution of this book without permission is a theft of the author's intellectual property. If you would like permission to use material from the book (other than for review purposes), please contact permissions@hbgusa.com. Thank you for your support of the author's rights.

Little, Brown Spark
Hachette Book Group
1290 Avenue of the Americas, New York, NY 10104
littlebrownspark.com

First Edition: December 2019

Little Brown Spark is an imprint of Little, Brown and Company, a division of Hachette Book Group, Inc. The Little, Brown Spark name and logo are trademarks of Hachette Book Group, Inc.

The publisher is not responsible for websites (or their content) that are not owned by the publisher.

The Hachette Speakers Bureau provides a wide range of authors for speaking events. To find out more, go to hachettespeakersbureau.com or call (866) 376-6591.

ISBN 978-0-316-52965-5 (hc) / 978-0-316-42638-1 (large print)
LCCN 2019948616

10 9 8 7 6 5 4 3 2 1

LSC-C

Printed in the United States of America

For my wife and best friend, Chelsea, who is the love of my life, and my father God, without whom none of this would have been possible

Contents

PART II

WHAT COLLAGEN CAN DO FOR YOU

PART III

THE COLLAGEN DIET PLAN

THE
COLLAGEN
DIET

The Missing Link to Modern Health

There are personal crises that stop you in your tracks, and there are others that spur you to search for answers and strive to make your life—and the lives of others—better. My mom's second cancer diagnosis was the latter.

Those of you who have read my books and follow my YouTube, Instagram, and Facebook videos know the story: I was in my mid-twenties and finishing up my training as a doctor when I received a tearful call from my mom. She had survived a tough bout of breast cancer when I was thirteen, and ever since her treatment, she'd struggled with her health. She was fatigued, depressed, and had hypothyroidism. The vibrant, athletic woman I'd known in my youth had become a shadow of her former self. In fact, her diminishment— a result of the medications she'd taken to fight off breast cancer—was the reason I had decided to go into the medical field. In the years following her diagnosis, I became determined to understand the causes of ill health and find better ways to address them—ones that didn't leave you with long-term symptoms that undermine your ability to live a full and fulfilling life.

I was immersed in this quest when I picked up the phone and heard my mom's tearful voice. She told me that her doctor had found a tumor in her lung. Her words broke my heart. Anyone who has heard a loved one utter the words "I have cancer" knows what a gut punch it is. It brings you to your knees. But as a health care practitioner, I was more prepared for it than I had been as a child. I'd been studying functional and integrative medicine and had learned a lot since my mom had faced her first cancer diagnosis. I recognized that this crisis was a call for me to step up and help. I knew that making some super-healthy tweaks to my mom's diet and lifestyle could bolster her ability to fight the disease. But I also knew that if I wanted to give my mom the kind of guidance she'd need to beat this illness once and for all, I would have to learn a lot more— and quickly.

From that day on, I made it my mission to read everything I could about food and healing. I learned about the ketogenic diet and its ability to reduce the corrosive effects of high blood sugar, insulin, and inflammation, allowing the body's innate healing mechanisms to step forward and take over. I investigated the healing properties of herbs and spices, which contain thousands of compounds that bolster the body's ability to fight disease. Studying Chinese and Ayurvedic medicine led me to a trove of medical wisdom that is used successfully in many parts of the world but is sadly underutilized in modern American health care. And I learned about bone broth, which contains key amino acids (the building blocks of proteins) that are absent in the types of muscle-meat protein most of us consume today.

Together, my mom and I carefully crafted a diet and lifestyle that would allow her to tackle her new health challenge from every angle: physically, emotionally, and spiritually. She ate a nutrient-dense diet of whole foods rich in antioxidants — foods like wild-caught salmon, leafy greens, mushrooms, and berries — and healing spices like turmeric. She also drank lots and lots of bone broth, which contains beneficial compounds that improved her energy, sleep, and ability to properly digest the rest of the food she was eating. After nine months on the protocol we designed, she beat cancer — without the use of dangerous drugs or toxic radiation treatments. Today, not only is my mom cancer-free, she is truly thriving. Her chronic fatigue, her thyroid problems, and her depression are gone. She's as healthy as she was before her first cancer diagnosis. She has, blessedly, returned to her old self.

My days and nights of intensive research paid off in a spectacular way that defied my mom's doctors' expectations—and they led me down promising new avenues of healing I've continued to explore as a functional medicine doctor to this day. One of the most exciting things I stumbled on during that time was bone broth and, more important, *collagen*, the powerhouse protein it contains. I've been studying this remarkable substance ever since.

Collagen is most famous for being a critical building block of healthy skin, so you may recognize it from the labels of beauty products. But its importance for health is far more than skin-deep. Collagen is the most abundant protein in the body. It's found in skin, nails, bone, cartilage, tendons, muscles, the gut lining, the disks that cushion your vertebrae, blood vessels, and the outer layer of your organs. Because it's woven into so many tissues, it plays a vital role in countless aspects of your health. In fact, new research is demonstrating that collagen and the compounds it contains may help regenerate new tissue, aid in gut repair, boost your immune system, and even increase your life span.

Based on my research, I believe it's *the* unsung hero of anti-aging medicine. It can help you

- avoid the aches and pains of aging
- stave off wrinkles and sagging skin
- heal persistent gastrointestinal issues or food sensitivities
- build your immune system, strengthening your resistance to cold and flu bugs

- maintain healthy nails and hair
- bolster the strength of your bones and muscles

I've scoured the scientific literature on this remarkable substance, uncovering study after study that confirms its benefits and points toward its untapped potential. At the same time, I've been blown away by the effects of collagen on the hundreds of patients, friends, and loved ones to whom I've recommended it. I've encouraged patients to consume collagen-rich smoothies and, in some cases, to follow a bone broth cleanse (during which they eat mostly bone broth), to help support healthy joints, ligaments, tendons, skin, and digestion. And just like my mom, these patients started feeling better.

But the thing that truly persuaded me of collagen's immense healing power was experiencing it firsthand. I've always had lots of energy. But several years after my mom's second battle with cancer, I found myself wiped out by fatigue and experiencing erratic bowel habits, alternating between constipation and loose stool. At first, I chalked up my symptoms to stress and overwork, the lifestyle conditions we tend to blame for all our inexplicable symptoms. And the theory made sense. I was putting in more than seventy hours each week treating patients and building DrAxe.com. I struggled to relieve my symptoms until I visited an acupuncturist who told me the root of the problem lay in my gut.

I'd already learned about leaky gut syndrome—a condition in which toxins, microbes, and undigested proteins like gluten are allowed to pass from the intestines into the bloodstream because the collagen-rich barrier designed to keep them inside the gut has become too permeable—and I knew that a healthy, anti-inflammatory diet was the best way to cure it.* But my diet was already chock-full of nutritious foods, with lots of inflammation-fighting veggies. The one thing I was missing, I realized, was collagen. I went from drinking bone broth only sporadically to consuming several cups on a daily basis. I focused on supporting my body's overall collagen production by eating chicken and salmon skin and consuming more vitamin C and red veggies, like tomatoes and beets, which contain lycopene, a substance that shores up collagen. And I began putting heaping scoops of powdered collagen in my morning smoothies. Over the course of several months my symptoms diminished, then went away completely.

Now I'm here to share what I've learned with you. We've ignored collagen for too long—and at our own peril. I wrote *The Collagen Diet* to change that. My goal is to help you learn how to take advantage of this valuable yet overlooked protein so you, too, can reap

---

* Leaky gut can be caused by antibiotics, which kill off both good and bad bacteria in your digestive tract, as well as by a lack of exposure to the microbes in dirt, where health-promoting soil-based organisms thrive; my book *Eat Dirt* offers an in-depth look at the problem and how to treat it.

its innumerable youth-preserving benefits. My approach is based on leading-edge science and offers a safe, effective way to restore your vitality, balance your hormones, and give your body the precise mix of key ingredients it needs to fortify collagen production for the long term. By the time you finish this book, you'll have a complete understanding of what collagen is, why it's so deeply critical for healthy aging, and how to use it to improve your health and well-being.

In Part I, we'll cover the collagen basics—everything you need to know about this underappreciated substance. I'll break down the science behind how collagen works and explain in clear, easy-to-understand language what collagen does for us, why it's so important as we age, and the many ways we can keep our levels high, from practical approaches, like exercise and diet, to cutting-edge theories on supporting stem cell production.

In Part II, we delve into the specific ways that collagen benefits us, like improving our appearance and gut function, eliminating pain, and resetting hormones—just to name a few. By the time you've finished this section, you'll see how diverse and important collagen is for your overall health and the dramatic impact it can have on everything from your daily functioning to your life span.

In Part III, I provide two step-by-step diet plans—a 3-day collagen cleanse and a 28-day collagen diet—that make it easy to apply what you've learned to your busy life. To help you make collagen a sustainable part of your diet, I've also included seventy-two delicious recipes designed to encourage your body's collagen production and give your skin, bones, gut, muscles, tendons, and blood vessels optimal amounts of this rejuvenating ingredient, so they will continue to function effectively and efficiently.

I'm grateful you've picked up this book, and I'm eager to share with you everything I've learned about how collagen can help you look and feel your best by supporting your body from the inside out. I swear by my collagen-rich diet. It supports my joints, helps me recover faster from the wear and tear of exercise, protects my digestive system, and keeps my body strong, flexible, and fit. And if you read this book and follow its collagen-boosting plan, I know you'll experience these benefits as well.

PART I

The Truth about Collagen

CHAPTER 1

The Essential Nutrient That Disappeared from Our Diets

Why Embracing This Ancient Dietary Staple Can Restore Your Health

We live in an era of unprecedented abundance. The food supply in the United States contains about 3,750 calories per person, per day. That's a thousand calories more than we consumed daily just two hundred years ago, according to the U.N. Food and Agricultural Organization, and far more than any of us needs. (Women require 2,000 calories, on average, and men 2,500.) Our ancient ancestors, who had to hunt wild game and gather berries to scrape together enough calories to feed their families, would undoubtedly be astonished by our effortless access to sustenance. And *envious.*

But here's the paradox: Despite the availability of food, many of us are plagued by surprisingly poor health. Nearly half of the people in the United States suffer from chronic conditions like diabetes, joint pain, heart disease, osteoporosis, gastrointestinal problems, inflammation, and cancer, undermining their ability to participate fully in daily activities and often cutting short their lives. Odds are, at least a handful of people you care about are affected by one or more of these persistent health problems. And the situation is likely to get worse, since most of these conditions become more prevalent with age—and our population is rapidly graying. Ten thousand people in the United States will turn sixty-five every day from now through the end of 2029, according to the Pew Research Center. The scope of the looming problem is mind-boggling. And here's what makes it even more tragic: Chronic health conditions can be traced, in large part, to our modern diet.

Food is called sustenance for a reason. It is meant to *sustain* us—not only to provide fuel for our bodies but also to heal them, to give us the nutrients we need to look and feel our best, and to provide us with ample energy to face the demands of our increasingly stressful lives. But here's the catch: We need to eat the *right* foods. And that's the problem we're facing now. The two "staples" of the typical Western diet, sugar and refined carbs, fill our bellies but shortchange our health. By providing largely empty calories, they pack on pounds, undermine our bodies' ability to function on a cellular level, fuel inflammation, and increase our risk of every single chronic condition that's rampant today.

We no longer live with chronic hunger or the persistent threat of starvation, as our ancestors did. But we are starved for true nourishment. A variety of studies over the past decade have found that many of us don't get enough calcium, potassium, fiber, folic acid, magnesium, iron, and vitamins A, C, and E—nutrients that are indispensable for building strong muscles, bones, blood vessels, skin, and immune systems. Other compounds that were plentiful in our ancestors' diets, like phosphorus, silicon, glucosamine, and sulfur, are missing from our everyday meals as well.

But there's a lesser-known substance that's notably absent from the typical Western diet—one that I believe can help us reverse our spiraling health issues and give all of us the best shot at a long, robust, active life. It's called collagen. It's the most abundant protein in the body, and a growing database of research shows it is vital for the structural integrity and healthy, long-term functioning of our bodies.

Our ancestors' diets were rich in collagen. Today, we consume almost none. But thanks to recent research showing that it can do everything from regenerating new tissue to bolstering your immune system, it's finally getting its due. I'm a huge fan of collagen. And I believe that by the time you've finished this book, you'll understand why—and you will be, too.

MEET THE INGREDIENT THAT JUST MIGHT CHANGE YOUR LIFE

Collagen is a strong, springy, fibrous substance that is woven into dozens of your body's tissues. It's responsible in large part for the firmness and elasticity of your skin, the strength of your nails and bones, and the pliability of your cartilage, tendons, muscles, gut lining, and blood vessels. It even encases your organs. On a functional level, collagen gives you flexibility and strength, allows your joints to move fluidly without aches and pains, and plays a role in everything from wound healing to gut health to cardiac health. It's the glue that holds you together. Indeed, the word *collagen* is derived from the Greek word for glue, *kolla*.

There are sixteen different types of collagen, but about 90 percent of the collagen in your body is either type I, II, or III—or some combination of the three. (I'll explain each type in the next chapter.) Those three predominant types share the same molecular structure—a woven rope–like shape known as a triple-stranded helix, which gives them their strength and flexibility.

Because it plays a vital role in so many diverse aspects of health, adding collagen to your diet is one of the best ways to fight off both the visible and invisible signs of aging and keep you feeling vibrant as the years tick by. For instance, a recent study published in the journal *Nutrients* looked at the effects of oral collagen supplementation on the skin of aging mice, a reasonable stand-in for human skin. (Studies that rely on taking widespread biopsies are often performed in mice instead of humans, for obvious reasons.) After eight weeks, not only did their skin have more collagen, but its ability to repair frayed collagen fibers had improved, its antioxidant enzymes were more active, and the skin itself was firmer.[1] It changed the tissue quantitatively and qualitatively, according to the researchers, effectively turning back the clock and making the skin's structure and appearance years younger.

As you get older, it becomes increasingly vital to get this substance from your diet. Here's why: In your mid-twenties, your body's natural collagen production begins to decline at a rate of about 1 percent per year — a drop-off that accelerates in your forties and fifties. By the time you reach your early fifties, you produce roughly 30 percent less natural collagen than you did in your twenties.

Waning collagen is a normal part of the aging process, but it is fueled by certain lifestyle habits, including sun exposure (ultraviolet radiation damages the skin's collagen-building cells), smoking, stress, poor gut health, consuming too much sugar, and inflammation (which often stems from poor diet and lifestyle habits). Molecules of sugar, for instance, form what's known as "advanced glycation end products," or AGEs, which can attach to the collagen and elastin in your skin, causing wrinkles and loss of elasticity and putting you at risk for inflammation-related skin conditions like acne and rosacea.

As a result, it's critical to replenish this diminishing source of youth and vitality, and the most important way to do that is with food. But the typical Western diet has been largely stripped of collagen. Every time you remove the skin from a chicken breast or put the tendinous gristle in the dog's bowl, you're throwing away an opportunity to bolster and sustain your body's collagen. And, as you'll learn in the coming pages, those are just two examples of the opportunities you're almost surely missing to bolster your body's collagen and take advantage of its regenerative effects.

There's no medical test to gauge how much collagen you have, but, honestly, you don't need one. It's easy to recognize when this fundamental substance is becoming dangerously low. Collagen deficiency makes itself known through

- Arthritis and joint pain. As you lose collagen-rich cartilage, achy joints become more common.
- Wrinkles, cellulite, and sagging skin. Collagen makes up 75 to 80 percent of skin. Without collagen to provide structure, skin sags and dimples.
- More frequent cuts and abrasions. Thinning skin is more vulnerable to daily wear and tear.

- Slower wound healing. As a glue-like substance, collagen helps the skin knit together.
- Hair loss. Collagen supports hair growth.
- Brittle nails. Collagen plays a role in nail growth and strength.
- Smaller, weaker muscles. Found in muscle tissue, collagen plays a role in muscle growth.
- Decreased bone density. There's actually more collagen than calcium in your bones!
- Gastrointestinal problems, like loose stool, gas, and bloating. As the protective, collagen-rich lining in your digestive tract thins, these symptoms become more common.
- Immune issues. Collagen supports your gut lining, and 70 percent of your immune system is housed in your gut.
- Chronic inflammation. Collagen contains glycine, an essential amino acid that's a powerful anti-inflammatory and helps protect the mucus lining of the gut.
- Food sensitivities. As the gut lining deteriorates due to collagen depletion, you're more likely to develop symptoms from eating foods that didn't bother you before.
- Heart problems. When the collagen in the lining of your arteries begins to degrade,

your arteries, which carry blood from your heart to your tissues, become less supple—a serious risk factor for heart disease and high blood pressure.

By getting enough collagen in your diet, you can prevent—and treat—many of these problems. Here's one example: In 2018, German researchers reported on the results of a study looking at collagen and bone loss. For the trial, they enrolled postmenopausal women whose bones were thinning. Some of the women consumed 5 grams of a collagen supplement every day for a year, while the others were given a placebo. After twelve months, the collagen group had significantly greater bone mineral density in their spines and the top of their femurs (the bone most associated with broken hips), while the placebo group's bones had become more fragile.[2]

I'm always wary when someone tells me a single substance has such broad and diverse effects, and frankly, you should be, too. But there's a simple explanation for why collagen can and does have an impact on so many different parts of your body: Like an invisible suit of protective armor, it's woven into a multitude of tissues, from the outermost layer of your skin to the innermost layer of your blood vessels.

Everywhere it's found, it serves to strengthen, fortify, build, and renew tissue at a cellular level. It's one of our best defenses against the ravages of age—and a powerful weapon for strengthening whole-body health and wellness. I've been recommending collagen to patients, friends, and family for the past decade and have seen remarkable examples of improved health and healing.

For instance, in 2018, my dear friend and colleague Jordan Rubin and I debuted a program called the Multi Collagen Makeover, which contains many of the same components as the *Collagen Diet* plan. As the program took off, dozens of participants sent us revealing feedback. As Debbie Fong, one participant, said, "I'm on day 21, and I feel like I'm reversing in age. I'll be sixty at the end of this year and I can see all the physical changes on the outside, so I can only imagine what it's doing on the inside of my body. My face glows now, and my skin is getting firmer. The bags under my eyes are diminishing, and the drooping under my eyelids is disappearing. My jawline is starting to reappear. Totally amazing!"

A growing body of research supports that type of anecdotal experience. Indeed, a 2019 review of the literature published in the *Journal of Drugs in Dermatology* concluded that oral collagen supplements increase the elasticity, hydration, and density of aging skin's collagen-rich dermis (the layer that determines, in large part, whether your skin is smooth or wrinkled)—all without any adverse side effects.[3]

New studies in this burgeoning field are revealing additional uses for collagen all the time. For instance, collagen is now being combined with stem cells to help regenerate knee and shoulder cartilage in those with injuries and arthritis. And resorbable forms of the substance are being used to dress oral wounds and promote dental healing.

In the coming chapters, I'll explain in detail the exciting studies on collagen and their results, which show it can improve the health of your skin, gut, joints, and more. But first, it's important for you to know a bit more about this substance so you'll better understand why it can have such powerful effects.

EVERYTHING OLD IS NEW AGAIN

Although collagen is on its way to becoming the "it" dietary ingredient (especially in supplement form), it's far from new. This humble protein formed the backbone of our ancient ancestors' diets, which were made up of wild meats and bone broth as well as vegetables, berries, herbs, and spices. In the days when food was scarce, humans used every edible part of the animal. They brewed collagen-rich broth from the bones, tendons, and cartilage of fish, chicken, and beef, and they routinely ate organ meats, ligaments, and tendons, all of which are teeming with life-giving collagen. As it turns out, their thrifty approach to food use may have offered them protection against some of the most common ailments that plague many of us today.

Take arthritis. This public health menace affects an estimated *54 million to 91 million* adults in the United States (the higher number includes people who haven't received an official diagnosis), causing chronic pain and forcing nearly half of sufferers to limit their daily activity. However, when researchers from Harvard and several other universities recently compared skeletons from modern people to those of hunter-gatherers and early farmers—skeletons that were as many as six thousand years old—as well as bones from the nineteenth and early twentieth centuries, they found that knee osteoarthritis is at least twice as common today as it was in prehistoric and early industrial times.[4]

All of the skeletons were from people who were fifty or older, and the researchers controlled for age, body mass index, and other confounding factors. Even so, osteoarthritis affected just 6 to 8 percent of the prehistoric samples and those from the 1800s and early 1900s, while skeletons from the 1900s to early 2000s showed a rate of 16 percent. And that's lower than the 23 percent the Centers for Disease Control reports.[5] Moreover, it is estimated that by 2040 nearly 26 percent of U.S. adults will be afflicted by the condition.

While the relatively recent rise in obesity has undoubtedly played a role in the uptick, weight only explains a fraction of the increase, according to the researchers' calculations. Their conclusion: In order to prevent this debilitating condition, we should try to adhere more closely to the physical activity and dietary patterns of our early ancestors. And here's what our ancestors ate: veggies, berries, herbs, and collagen, collagen, collagen.

Our forefathers' high-collagen diets may also have protected them from common gastrointestinal conditions that afflict far too many people today. In a study published in *Nature Communications,* researchers analyzed the gut bacteria of the Hadza, a foraging tribe in western Tanzania.[6] The Hadza, who still live entirely on wild game, roots, and berries, just as our ancient ancestors did, not only have radically different gut bacteria from the average modern urbanite but also have zero incidence of irritable bowel syndrome and Crohn's disease.

Studies like these support the intriguing idea that collagen has historically played an important role in human health. Although our ancestors originally consumed the collagen-rich parts of animals for practical reasons—when food is scarce it makes sense to get every ounce of nutrition you can out of every food source—they undoubtedly benefited physically from the approach. And there's ample evidence that a number of cultures around the world learned the value of this substance and began to utilize it as a cure for a variety of ailments. Indeed, collagen has featured heavily in traditional healing modalities around for world for centuries.

In China, for instance, people have been using gelatin made from boiled-down donkey skin for thousands of years to keep their skin looking young and healthy. When you simmer the collagen-packed bones of an animal, as you do when you make bone broth, they eventually break down into gelatin. In other words, like bone broth, gelatin is rich in collagen; it's just in a different form.

In Traditional Chinese Medicine (TCM), healers also mix donkey skin gelatin, or *ejiao,* with a variety of herbs typically used in TCM to increase energy, improve sleep, and bolster circulation. There are even references dating back as far as the first century BCE to people in China and Japan using gelatin as a hemostatic agent to promote blood-clotting for everything from nosebleeds to internal bleeding. It's so effective that hospitals to this day use a gelatin-based substance to promote clotting.

In the twelfth century, Moses Maimonides, the Egyptian Jewish physician, prescribed chicken broth made from the bones of chicken to treat colds—another remedy that is still in use today. (Canned chicken soups contain collagen, but they're often loaded with sodium and preservatives. You're better off making your own.) And over the years, gelatin from a variety of sources has been used to treat bone and muscle weaknesses as well as digestive problems. In the early twentieth century, for instance, the well-known nutritionist Francis Pottenger Jr. prescribed gelatin for a range of digestive complaints, including ulcers, heartburn, and vomiting. In other words, collagen has long been a staple of medicine and healing.

HOW TO EMBRACE A COLLAGEN-RICH DIET

Although the idea of nose-to-tail eating — consuming every conceivable part of an animal — is an underground trend in the United States today, it's not the way most of us eat. There are a number of contemporary cultures, however, that never turned their backs on this crucial practice.

In Alaska, Canada, and Russia, for instance, *muktuk,* made from the collagen-rich blubber and skin of whales, is a staple of the Inuit diet. And head cheese, popular for hundreds of years in Europe and elsewhere, is a gelatinous cold cut made from the head of a calf or pig, along with other body parts, like the tongue, feet, and heart. In fact, most traditional diets worldwide, from Asia to South America to Europe, rely on healthy quantities of collagen.

If you read the words *head cheese* and think, "Yuck!" you're not alone. I believe some traditional collagen-rich foods are worth trying for their health value and unique flavor, but rest assured: there are plenty of ways to get more collagen in your diet without eating tongue or brain.

One of my favorites is to make bone broth by simmering the bones of chickens, cows, or fish in a soup pot with other healthy ingredients, like carrots, onion, celery, and bay leaves. Bone broth is a staple of the daily diet my wife, Chelsea, and I consume, and I recommend it to everyone. If you make one change to your dietary routine, this should be it. Bone broth is nutrient-dense, easy to digest, health-promoting, and absolutely delicious. Moreover, you'll derive different benefits depending on the bones you use. Here's a quick breakdown of the collagen-related qualities of each type:

- Bovine collagen, from the bones, skin, cartilage, and tendons of cows, is largely made of types I and III, two of the three most abundant collagen types in your body. It provides you with a healthy dose of the amino acids glycine and proline (in the following chapter I'll explain more about these amino acids), as well as the all-star joint-protecting substances, glucosamine and chondroitin. It's a valuable ally for building muscle and promoting your body's own collagen production.
- Chicken collagen, from the bones, skin, and gristle of chicken, is rich in type II collagen, and as a result is best for building cartilage. It also provides chondroitin sulfate and glucosamine sulfate, both of which

are also great for joint health and work synergistically with collagen.

■ Fish collagen, from the bones and skin of fish, is easy for your body to absorb and is mostly type I, the single most common form of collagen in your body. Consuming fish collagen can provide widespread benefits; it can improve the structural integrity of everything from your joints and skin to your vital organs, blood vessels, gastrointestinal tract, and bones.

■ Egg collagen is found in the membrane inside the shells of eggs. It's mostly type I but has traces of types III, IV, and X. It provides glucosamine, chondroitin, hyaluronic acid (another hot substance in the anti-aging realm that we'll learn more about later), and various other amino acids that benefit connective tissue, wound healing, muscle building, and joint pain and stiffness. Of course, it's hard to eat eggshell membrane, so this type of collagen is mostly found in supplements.

Bone broth is a simple, tasty way to boost your daily collagen consumption, but it's far from the only one. You can also use protein powder made from bone broth in a variety of recipes, from soups to smoothies to sauces. You can start eating the skin on fish and chicken. And you can eat the organ meats of animals, which are high in collagen. Simpler still, you can take supplements that contain hydrolyzed collagen. These are collagen peptides that have undergone a process known as hydrolysis to break them down into shorter chains of proteins. Studies show that hydrolized collagen supplements can have the same positive effects on your health as whole collagen. Or you can eat gelatin, as more and more athletes are doing to heal injuries and joint pain—which delivers the same benefits as hydrolyzed collagen.

As you begin to increase your collagen intake, it's important to take a look at the rest of your diet, too, to ensure that you're consuming foods that limit inflammation and support collagen production, like delicious vegetables and nutrient-packed herbs, and avoiding those, like sugar and carbs, that diminish it. And you also might need to tweak your lifestyle to reduce inflammation, a collagen killer. It's important to get plenty of sleep, for instance, to exercise regularly, and to reduce stress, which triggers us to reach for foods high in sugar and simple carbs. In the coming chapters I'll lay out simple strategies for making incremental changes that will help you feel a whole lot better and help you take full advantage of collagen's power.

I believe that collagen is the true missing link to modern health. I've recommended it to hundreds of patients, and the transformations they've made to their health and physical appearance have convinced me that we all need to embrace this vital element of ancient nutrition. When we don't get enough of the beneficial compounds found in collagen-rich foods, the tissues in our bodies break down more quickly and we suffer the consequences—from hindered mobility to deficient digestion. In order to achieve sustainable wellness that lasts a lifetime, we must return to a collagen-rich diet, which served our ancestors so well. It's time to reclaim this age-old tradition and restore and rejuvenate our vitality.

CHAPTER 2

The Smart New Way to Think about Dietary Protein

Why You Likely Have an Amino Acid Imbalance — And How Collagen Can Help

If you've ever picked up a weight-loss book, browsed a health blog, or tried a fad diet, you're undoubtedly familiar with the word *protein*. Protein is one of three "macronutrients" in the human diet, along with fat and carbohydrates. Most popular weight-loss plans today advise eating more protein — and for good reason: It is not only the single most important ingredient for building and maintaining your muscles, organs, tissues, and cells; it's also present in foods that are satiating, so it keeps you full longer. And since dietary protein builds muscle, the premier calorie-burning tissue in your body, it bolsters your metabolism and is critical for reaching your ideal weight and shape. Collagen is one important type of protein, and it's largely missing, as I've mentioned, from modern diets, because it is found in parts of the animals that we typically discard—the bones, skin, tendons, and cartilage.

Your body contains protein, too. About 17 percent of your tissues are made up of protein, and collagen is the most abundant type of protein in the body. This multitasking workhorse helps keep your gut healthy, plumps up your skin, cushions your joints, and plays a role in everything from immunity to hormone balance. Simply put, protein, including collagen protein, is vital to the healthy functioning of nearly every physical aspect of your body. It's not a stretch to say that without protein, life wouldn't exist.

But without amino acids, protein wouldn't exist. Amino acids are the building blocks of protein, including collagen, and they combine in a variety of ways to form a huge range of tissues. There are twenty-one different kinds of amino acids, and together they're responsible for building and repairing nearly every part of your body. Nine of them are considered "essential," which means you can't manufacture them internally. Since you literally can't survive without them, they *must* come from your diet. They're found in the most abundant quantities in meat, eggs, and dairy, but they're also in nuts, seeds, grains, vegetables, and mushrooms—which means it's vital to eat some of these foods.

But here's the critical factor that has been missing from that equation for far too long: In order for your body to function at its best, you need an amino acid *balance.* For the past one hundred years or more, our culture has focused predominantly on muscle meat as our main source of protein — foods like chicken breast, lamb chops, filets, and skinless fish — and turned its back on a variety of healing, collagen-rich parts of the animal, like skin, bones, and cartilage. But these discarded animal tissues contain other important but nonessential amino acids found in only small quantities in muscle meats.

In ignoring these tissues, we've created a nationwide epidemic of amino acid imbalance, meaning our ratio of essential to nonessential amino acids is badly out of whack. Amino acid imbalance isn't an acute health problem, like cancer. But make no mistake: It's a slow killer. As the years pass, it quietly, incrementally, almost unnoticeably undermines and erodes your health. But there's an easy fix. By adding collagen to your diet, you can turn it around.

WHY THE AMINO ACIDS IN COLLAGEN ARE SO IMPORTANT

The majority of the collagen in your body is made up of interwoven chains of important amino acids: glycine, proline, and, depending on the exact type of collagen, a third amino acid, often arginine, or hydroxyproline, an amino acid precursor. The amino acids in collagen are known as "conditionally essential." You can survive without them, but when you're under stress or battling an illness, they're essential, according to the National Library of Medicine. And who isn't under stress? Our nonstop 24/7 culture means most of us need these conditionally essential amino acids all the time—possibly more than ever in human history.

For most of us, these conditionally essential amino acids in collagen are actually essential. But if you're not consciously making an effort to consume collagen-rich foods, like bone broth, gelatin, and the skin of chicken and fish, your body is being largely deprived of these vital building blocks.

And that nutritional void can have ramifications for your health. For instance, muscle meat contains an essential amino acid known as methionine, which plays several key roles in the body—it promotes the production of glutathione, for instance, which is known as the body's master antioxidant. But methionine also has a dark side. Dozens of studies in rodents have shown that by decreasing methionine in their diets (it is found in the highest quantities in beef, cereal, dairy, eggs, and brazil nuts), they consistently live 10 to 20 percent longer. In other words, getting too much methionine can shorten your life.

Although long-term methionine restriction studies are impossible in humans for ethical and logistical reasons, laboratory research on human cells shows a similar effect on life span: Low methionine equals longer life. And there are other dangers of methionine. A study published in the *Journal of Clinical Endocrinology & Metabolism* found that when obese people restricted methionine, their ability to burn stubborn body fat increased.[7] And a study in *Nutrition, Metabolism & Cardiovascular Diseases* found that high dietary methionine intake increased the risk of acute cardiovascular events like heart attacks in middle-aged men.[8]

One reason methionine can adversely affect your health is because it raises blood levels of another amino acid, homocysteine—and homocysteine not only increases the risk of diabetes and heart disease but also may accelerate aging.

But here's why adding collagen to your diet and creating a healthier balance of amino acids is so important: When you consume collagen, the body breaks it down into its constituent amino acids—and glycine, one of the main amino acids in all types of collagen, not only reduces homocysteine levels in the blood after a high-protein meal but also helps the liver metabolize excess methionine, reducing its negative effects on health and life span. In other words, by consuming a little collagen every day, you rein in the damage caused by a muscle-meat-heavy diet. Eating collagen provides amino acid balance.

The amino acids in collagen have a variety of other vitally important effects. Here's a quick overview of the latest findings on the two key collagen-related amino acids:

■ *Glycine* is high in the collagen found in your skin, connective tissue, joints, and muscles. This all-star amino acid supports cognitive performance and central nervous system functioning by regulating nutrients that the brain and nerves use for energy. It also balances electrolyte levels, like calcium, chloride, and potassium, thereby promoting better regulation of nerve impulses. In the body, glycine helps break down fat, allowing it to be used as energy by cells.

But there are additional reasons it is quickly becoming recognized as a wonder substance. A number of recent studies, for instance, have shown that glycine can help you sleep. In one paper published in *Sleep and Biological Rhythms*, researchers gave people struggling with insomnia 3 grams of glycine before bed. The study subjects said they slept better and felt less tired the next day—and objective analysis confirmed it; the time it took them to fall asleep and to drop into slow-wave sleep was shortened.[9] That's hopeful news for the 25 percent or more of people who suffer from insomnia each year. Many sleep medications have dangerous side effects. Glycine has none.

The most exciting new research reveals that glycine appears to fight aging on the mitochondrial level. As we get older, our mitochondria, the tiny, energy-producing organelles inside our cells, develop defects. That's a key reason we can't run as far or as fast at age fifty as we could at twenty; it's also the reason we get more fatigued from a long day at work as we age. But preliminary laboratory research has shown that adding glycine to a culture containing cells from a ninety-seven-year-old person transformed the aged mitochondria. The respiratory defects the mitochondria had accrued over the years disappeared, and the tiny organelles' functional capabilities were restored.[10]

That finding dovetails with promising new research in animals. Glycine supplementation has been shown to increase life span in rats, mice, and *C. elegans,* a tiny wormlike creature that's commonly used in anti-aging research. Researchers speculate that glycine might help extend life by increasing glutathione, which, as I mentioned above, is known as the body's master antioxidant. Glutathione heals damage to cells' DNA and mitochondria caused by free radicals — unstable molecules that, left unchecked, can wreak havoc and accelerate aging and disease.

■ *Proline* is the other main component of collagen. In fact, the first stage of collagen synthesis begins with a three-dimensional strand known as procollagen — a collagen precursor — primarily made up of glycine and proline. One of proline's key responsibilities is helping form new protein in the body, including collagen and connective tissue, cartilage, skin, and the lining of the gut.

In addition, when you have a wound, proline swings into action to help it heal. Studies have found that levels of the substance at wound sites are at least 50 percent higher than plasma levels — and plasma is known for the key role it plays in healing. Other research has shown that proline is actively involved in every phase of the wound healing process, from stimulating the migration of cells to building new tissue. Proline is also an important component of healthy skin. As we age, our skin tends to get thinner, and as a result, more abrasion prone. But consuming a healthy amount of proline-containing collagen can help keep your skin strong, making it more impervious to everyday scratches and scrapes. There's even preliminary evidence that proline can reduce the appearance of cellulite by firming and tightening skin.

Finally, proline's ability to generate new tissue can benefit people who suffer from joint pain or gastrointestinal problems or are at increased risk of heart disease. And it can bolster metabolism and muscle mass, increasing energy output during physical activity, which makes it helpful for weight control.

Glycine and proline aren't the only two amino acids in collagen. Certain types contain glutamic acid, a precursor to glutamine, which performs a variety of important functions, like preventing anxiety and improving sleep, concentration, digestive health, immune system function, and energy. High glutamine levels encourage your body to produce nitrogen, which helps with wound healing and prevents muscle wasting (a common and often dire problem that tends to go hand in hand with aging) and joint pain. Arginine is also found in collagen, and new studies are revealing a variety of uses that you'll hear more about in Chapter 10. Turns out, it's critical for the health of your heart and arteries. It can improve circulation, reduce blood pressure, and strengthen the immune system.

WELCOME TO THE NEW IDEA OF AMINO ACID BALANCE

You already know that you should consume a range of vegetables, or "eat the rainbow," since each source, whether beets or brussels sprouts, contains unique vitamins and minerals that bolster your body in various ways. In my book *Keto Diet,* I explain why it's important to get a variety of types of fat in your diet as well. Research has shown, for instance, that a diet lacking in omega-3 fats and abundant in omega-6 fats can increase system-wide inflammation and put you at increased risk for inflammation-related diseases, like heart disease, chronic pain, diabetes, and cancer.

A balance of healthy fats is crucial to a healthy diet, but so is an appropriate balance of muscle-meat protein and collagen protein—and at this point, the average American diet is way off the mark. Most people get 95 percent or more of their protein from meat, eggs, dairy, and plant sources and 5 percent or less from collagen-rich sources, like bone broth, fish or chicken skin, organ meats, or gelatin. But since 30 percent of all protein in your body is collagen, you should aim to get 25 to 35 percent of your daily protein from collagen—maybe even as high as 50 percent for people over fifty-five or sixty, whose collagen levels are already diminished.

This way of thinking about protein is relatively new to nutritionists and will almost certainly be new to you. But it's important. Twelve years ago, very few of my patients had heard of omega-3 fats. Now, nearly every American knows what they are—and how critical they are for overall health. A decade down the road, the same will be true of dietary collagen. Everyone will understand the health value of adding collagen to their diets. That's why I'm delighted to introduce you to this concept. By reading this book, you are one of the first to be turned on to this under-the-radar health breakthrough!

If you're not eating a balanced protein diet—and by "balanced" I mean one that includes collagen—you're depriving your body of the raw materials it needs to maintain and sustain many of its most important tissues and functions. The amino acids in collagen not only support healthy collagen production but also complement and work synergistically with those found in our usual protein foods, like the muscle meat of beef, chicken, and fish. They're an essential part of the protein equation—and adding them to your diet can bolster your overall health and even your longevity.

A collagen deficiency can have health effects that

most doctors who aren't knowledgeable about nutrition will miss. Several years ago, I worked with a patient, Nicky, who was in her mid-twenties. She was superactive—a yoga instructor, who was also an enthusiastic CrossFit devotee. Even so, her joints were achy and painful, particularly her knees and wrists. She wasn't even thirty, and she was already suffering from pain so severe that she had to take a break from exercise and teaching, her main source of income. She told me that she consumed lots of veggies and fruit and quite a bit of protein—which, at first blush, sounds like a perfectly well-rounded diet. But because she was suffering from joint pain, I suspected she needed more collagen. She was busy and didn't have time to make bone broth, so I suggested she try using a couple of scoops of a collagen supplement in her morning smoothie, an excellent substitute for collagen-rich bone broth or organ meats. When I saw her two weeks later, she was all smiles. Her joints were feeling better, she told me. Within a month she was back to her usual intense level of daily exercise—and she has been able to maintain her activity without pain to this day.

RETHINKING YOUR DIETARY PROTEIN NEEDS

Protein is vital for your health. Every day, your body taps into its amino acid reserves to carry out numerous life-saving functions, from supporting digestion to supporting hormone and neurotransmitter production. Without enough protein in your diet, your body can't effectively repair damaged tissues or undertake the constant process of regeneration that keeps all your muscles and organs functioning properly. And dietary protein contributes to your amino acid reserves, a reservoir that you call upon every day.

As you read through the coming pages, keep in mind that certain stressors—processed foods, emotional stress, sleep deprivation, environmental pollution from cars, pesticides, smoking, and excessive alcohol consumption—deplete this crucial reservoir. Some are more controllable than others, but it's important to try to do what you can to maintain a physical environment that doesn't reduce your amino acid levels.

A great first step: Eat a clean diet, with the very best sources of protein, like grass-fed beef, lamb, and venison; pasture-raised chicken, turkey, and eggs; wild-caught fish and seafood; raw, organic dairy products; and plenty of bone broth. I realize these options can be expensive, sometimes prohibitively, so do the best you can within your means. I'm encouraging you to focus on clean protein not because it's trendy but because it can make a difference for your health. When animals aren't raised humanely, they tend to become sick and require the use of antibiotics, hormones, and chemicals, which wind up in the food supply—and in your body.

And keep in mind that you don't need enormous quantities of muscle-meat protein — just 0.36 gram per pound of body weight for the average adult. (Athletes and people who exercise strenuously every day need about double that amount.) That's about 46 grams if you weigh 130 pounds and 64 grams if you weigh 180. A three-ounce cooked chicken breast contains about 21 grams of protein.

The other thing that will make a difference is adding protein in the form of collagen to round out your amino acid intake. Here's one way I like to think about amino acid consumption: Imagine your body is a building. Traditional sources of protein, like steak or salmon, are the bricks — the big solid hunks that make up the majority of the structure. When you eat meat, the amino acids it contains help build new muscle, the brawny workhorse tissue in your body, and keep many of your body's systems functioning.

But if meat, eggs, and dairy are the bricks, collagen is the *mortar.* It holds the entire structure together and keeps it solid. It prevents the bricks from rubbing together and becoming eroded and askew. When you consume collagen, you reinforce your skin, cartilage, tendons, and ligaments, as well as the linings of various tissues, from your gut to your blood vessels. Mortar isn't more important than bricks. But without it, your structure is unstable and will begin to show signs of wear — and eventually collapse — far sooner than if you had maintained a solid level of mortar all along.

Amino acid balance is a new way of thinking about protein. And luckily there is a simple way to deal with this prevalent but largely unrecognized problem of protein imbalance. By adding healthy amounts of collagen to your diet you can bring your amino acid levels into a more wholesome equilibrium — a state that will give you the internal tools you need to fight aging and function optimally for the long term.

CHAPTER 3

The Cool New Breakthrough Science on Collagen

What It Is, Where It Is, and Why You Need Different Types

It's hard to believe there's one nutrient you can add to your diet that will help you sleep better at night, support healthy muscle tissue, and reverse many of the issues that crop up with aging. But collagen is an incredibly versatile substance. It *has* to be, since it's found in such disparate areas throughout the body. Think about it. Your skin is far different structurally from your bones, and cartilage is unlike muscles or ligaments or the lining of blood vessels. And yet collagen is woven into each one—and in some cases it makes up the bulk of the tissue.

How can a single substance assume so many diverse forms? The answer is simple: While this multipurpose tissue goes by a single name, its structure varies depending on where it is in the body. In fact, over the past ninety years or so, researchers have identified at least twenty-eight different types of collagen, as many as sixteen of which are embedded in the human body, where they offer structural support, serve as a protective barrier to ward off injuries and dangerous microbes, and allow us to maintain a strong, yet flexible, physique.

As I've said, getting more collagen in your diet is increasingly essential as you age and your collagen-dense tissues begin to experience wear and tear. Adding 20 to 50 grams of the substance to your daily diet can improve the health of your gut, skin, joints, hair, nails, immune system, vertebral disks, and blood vessels. But I don't want you to accept my recommendations at face value. I came to believe in collagen by understanding the research. It's important for you to understand it, too, so you'll be better equipped to make the best call for your own health. With that in mind, let's take a deeper look at what happens when you consume collagen—as well as at the most important types of collagen—and explore how the simple habit of getting more of each type in your daily diet can be a boon for your well-being and even add years to your life.

WHERE COLLAGEN IS FOUND — AND WHY IT CAN MAKE A REMARKABLE DIFFERENCE FOR YOUR HEALTH

When you're young, your body is, quite literally, a collagen-making machine. Starting at around age twenty-five, however, production begins a gradual decline. While you continue to manufacture the substance your whole life, you'll have a more robust yield, and avoid the problems that come with collagen deficiency, if you add the substance to your diet.

When you consume the skin on a chicken thigh or a scoop of a hydrolyzed collagen in your morning smoothie, your gut breaks it down into its key components: amino acids. Your body then uses those amino acids to rebuild your collagen-dense tissues. For instance, recent research has found peptides (short chains of amino acids) in the blood one hour after consuming less than 2 grams of collagen—and the quantity of peptides in the blood increases in a step-wise manner with higher and higher oral doses.[11] At the same time, when researchers traced radioactively labeled collagen peptides, they found evidence of the short amino acid chains in the skin, cartilage, and intestinal walls.[12] And a study in the *Journal of Cosmetic Dermatology* found that oral collagen supplements increased collagen density in the dermis, the collagen-containing layer of skin that lies just below the epidermis, or outer layer, after four weeks—and increased skin hydration after eight weeks.[13]

Here's how your body's internal collagen production plant works: Your connective tissue contains specialized cells known as fibroblasts. For the most part, this is where your body begins creating collagen. (Some cells in the skin and encasing the organs manufacture it as well.) The DNA in the nucleus of each fibroblast holds the specific recipe for putting together one type of collagen. Just as a car goes through a variety of stages as it makes its way through production, the complex assembly line of collagen production makes a series of stops within the cell itself. Along the way, immature amino acid groups are formed and undergo a process known as hydroxylation—essentially attaching hydrogen and oxygen to the amino acid strands to make the substance more stable. Hydroxylation requires vitamin C—another reason it's vitally important to make sure you get enough of this nutrient. (Scurvy, the most well-known collagen-deficiency disorder, develops in people who consume too little vitamin C; its symptoms include bleeding gums, weak blood vessels, and skin ulcers.)

Eventually, the characteristic braid-like triple helix strands are created. The fibroblast secretes these mature collagen strands into the area *outside* the cell, known as the extracellular matrix, or ECM. (We think of our tissues as being made up of cells, but a large portion of tissue volume is filled by the non-cell-based ECM; this intricate, dynamic network of large molecules, including collagen molecules, determines each tissue's physical properties and is constantly being remodeled and modified.)

In the ECM, the collagen strands are assembled into tough, flexible, three-dimensional collagen fibrils composed of differing sequences of amino acids—each of which gives rise to one of the sixteen different types of collagen. By the end of the process, every type of collagen possesses distinct properties that are perfectly tailored to the needs of the body part in which it will be used. The type of collagen in your bones, for instance, is more rigid, while that in your tendons is more flexible—cartilage is somewhere in between.

Although there are sixteen variations, six of them account for roughly 99 percent of your total collagen, and as a result they are the most important for your health and well-being. Here's what you need to know about each:

- Type I makes up more than 90 percent of the collagen in your body. These fibrils are remarkable in that they are capable of withstanding forceful stretching without breaking. Gram for gram, type I collagen is stronger than steel. It has to be, considering the types of tissues where it is used: skin, bones, tendons (which connect muscles with bones), ligaments (which connect bones and hold joints together), the supporting structures surrounding organs, the meniscus (the cartilage between the surface of some joints, including the knee), and the intervertebral disks that connect the bones of your vertebrae.

This tissue is truly remarkable. It literally holds us together. Anytime we run, jump, or lift, we place enormous force on our ligaments, tendons, and cartilage. We're able to avoid injury and move with ease thanks to type I collagen's superhero strength and elasticity.

Edible type I collagen is being studied for a number of potential uses in the health realm, particularly for the skin. I'll go into this fascinating research in more depth in Chapter 5, but here's an example of what scientists have discovered: A recent study in the *Journal of Aging Research & Clinical Practice* showed that consuming type I collagen peptides was more helpful than placebo for decreasing crow's-feet and increasing skin firmness in women ages forty-six to sixty-nine.[14] Oral type I collagen was also shown to hold potential for treating patients with cutaneous systemic sclerosis, a serious condition characterized by skin thickening that can also affect the organs and the lungs; in the study, researchers found that patients with late-phase disease had a significant reduction in their skin-thickness scores compared with those who received a placebo.[15]

And skin isn't the only tissue that benefits from this versatile protein. Daily type I collagen consumption has been shown to reduce pain in people with osteoarthritis, and a study in the medical journal *PLOS One* that looked at mice with injury-induced osteoarthritis found dose-dependent increases in cartilage in the injured joints as well as an increase in the number of healthy cartilage cells, known as chondrocytes.[16]

You can bolster your type I collagen intake by consuming foods rich in the substance, including bone broth (type I is found in beef bones and muscles), fish skin, and eggshell membrane.

- Type II primarily helps build cartilage, which is found in connective tissue. The health of your joints relies on cartilage, for instance, which is why type II collagen has been shown to be beneficial for preventing arthritis and other age-related joint pain. This spongelike tissue is also found in the inner core (known as the nucleus pulposus) of your intervertebral disks, so it plays a role in cushioning your spine and keeping it healthy and pain-free as well.

Evidence of its effectiveness has appeared in the scientific literature for years. For instance, in one trial a group of researchers compared the effectiveness of type II collagen with that of glucosamine and chondroitin in a group of patients with osteoarthritis of the knee. At the end of the ninety-day study, both groups improved; however, on every measure—including stiffness, physical function, and pain during daily activities—the participants who took collagen had a two to three times stronger response, a fascinating finding considering how many arthritis sufferers rely on glucosamine and chondroitin to ease their suffering. The researchers, who published the paper in the *International Journal of Medical Sciences,* concluded that subjects treated with type II collagen "showed significant enhancement in daily activities, suggesting an improvement in their quality of life."[17]

Likewise, there is evidence that consuming type II collagen for three months reduces joint pain and swelling in people with rheumatoid arthritis—and even reduces the time it takes those with the illness to walk about fifty feet.[18]

To increase your intake of type II collagen, eat more chicken skin and broth made from chicken, duck, or turkey bones, as well as collagen supplements that specifically contain type II.

■ Type III is found in skin and blood vessels and is a major component of the extracellular matrix, the delicate mesh-like tissue surrounding the organs, including the heart. In fact, the myocardial connective tissue that maintains the functional integrity of the heart is about 80 percent type I collagen and 20 percent type III—a common combination throughout the body.

Deficiencies in type III collagen have been linked in animal studies to a higher risk of ruptured blood vessels and even early death. The best sources of type III are the muscle and bones of cows (think: bone broth) and supplements; make sure they specify that they contain type III.

- Type IV plays a vital, unsung role in health. Because of the unique way its fibers link, it's more pliable than other types of collagen and can form sheets. As a result, it's found primarily in the basal lamina, a specialized type of extracellular matrix that can be structured in several ways—and is found in a variety of tissues throughout the body. Muscle fibers, for instance, are encased in basal lamina, which helps regenerate the tissue after injury; basal lamina can also sit underneath sheets of epithelial cells (which line the surfaces of your skin, organs, urinary tract, and blood vessels), where it provides support for the tissue, limits contact between epithelial cells and other types of cells, and acts as a filter that allows only water and small molecules to pass through; and the basal lamina can separate two sheets of cells, as it does in the kidneys, where it serves as a sort of molecular sieve, allowing only certain particles through.

The basal lamina is part of what's known as the basement membrane zone, thin, sheet-like structures that support cells in many tissues, including the inner ear, eye, and blood vessels, and help regulate cell behavior. The basement membrane zone is also essential for the development of embryos and new blood vessels.

In addition, type IV collagen is also vital for wound healing. German researchers analyzed sixty-two human skin wounds (including surgical wounds and stab wounds) and found type IV collagen helps knit the skin basement membrane zone together, allowing it to fully heal.[19] The best way to get type IV into your diet is through supplements; check the label to make sure yours contains it.

■ Type V is less prevalent but no less necessary than some of the other collagens. First isolated in the placenta, the organ that develops in a woman's uterus during pregnancy to provide oxygen and nutrients to the fetus, it has since been found throughout the body's connective tissue. Research shows type V is present in the cornea (where it makes up 15 to 20 percent of its total collagen), skin, uterus, kidneys, lungs, liver, pancreas, periodontal tissue that connects teeth to bones, and synovial membranes, the specialized connective tissue that lines the inner surface of joints. It's used to manufacture hair strands as well as cell membranes, the porous outer layer of every cell that holds its contents together and lets nutrients in while keeping pathogens and toxins out.

A deficiency of type V is associated with loss of corneal functioning in a connective-tissue disorder known as Ehlers-Danlos syndrome. You can get plenty of this nutrient by consuming beef bone broth or through supplements that specify that they contain it.

■ Type X is a bit of an outlier, because it's not associated with cartilage so much as bone. Indeed, it's integral to the process of what's known as endochondral ossification, the mechanism responsible for bone formation from conception through adolescence. The process begins when chondrocytes, the cells found in healthy cartilage, synthesize their characteristic extracellular matrix that's rich in type II collagen and other substances. The chondrocytes proliferate, promoting more matrix production. At a certain point, the chondrocytes stop multiplying and undergo maturation, secreting a new matrix containing type X collagen. That distinct type X-infused matrix then undergoes rapid calcification, becoming bone.

A similar process seems to occur throughout life as bone is continually remodeled—and the same mechanism swings into action to repair a broken bone. Indeed, a study of mice with bone fractures published in the *Journal of Cell Biochemistry* found that accelerated healing was associated with higher expression of a variety of substances, including type X and type II collagen.[20] Type X is found in eggshell membrane and chicken skin, as well as supplements that specifically say they contain it.

THE SEVEN SUBSTANCES THAT MAXIMIZE COLLAGEN PRODUCTION AND FUNCTION

Consuming a diet rich in collagen is the best way to replenish your body's diminishing supply. But to completely maximize your collagen growth and minimize collagen breakdown, there are seven essential substances that you also need to get from your diet—substances that will help you look and feel younger.

Known as collagen "cofactors," these key nutrients help your body synthesize proteins and lipids to form different tissues, especially cartilage. They can also help your body retain collagen and make it function more effectively. And they do a lot more. Cofactors tame rampant inflammation and reduce free radical damage, both of which are important for the health of your body's collagen-rich tissues. They support joint health, mobility, and flexibility. They help form the cartilage that surrounds your joints as well as the synovial fluid that provides lubrication to your joints. They aid in your ability to recover and benefit from exercise. And they support the health of your bones, gut, and immune system.

Here are the seven cofactors that are the most important:

- *Vitamin C.* I mentioned this legendary nutrient in the prior section and explained that it's vital to hydroxylation, the process by which collagen strands build stability. If you don't get enough vitamin C, your collagen production will slow and you'll suffer earlier and more severely from the problems associated with low collagen, like wrinkled skin, gut problems, achy joints, and lackluster nails and hair. Although the current dietary guidelines call for just 90 milligrams a day for men and 75 for women, I suggest you supplement the daily amount you get through diet by taking up to 1,000 milligrams of vitamin C-rich powders made from sources like amla berry, camu camu, acerola cherry, kakuda plum, baobab, and sea buckthorn.

- *Copper.* Getting a daily dose of this mineral will help activate lysyl oxidase, an enzyme that stabilizes collagen fibrils by building crosslinks with elastin, another protein that adds elasticity to connective tissue. Without this crosslinking, collagen doesn't mature properly, putting you at risk of weak bones, among other problems. Good sources of copper include beef liver, oysters, lobster, squid, and a variety of seeds and nuts, including sesame seeds, sunflower seeds, cashews, and almonds. Aim for 900 micrograms a day.

- *Zinc.* Consuming enough zinc is important because the mineral activates proteins essential for collagen synthesis as well as proteins that play a vital role in wound healing. Good sources of zinc include lamb, pumpkin seeds, grass-fed beef, garbanzo beans, cashews, kefir, mushrooms, spinach, and chicken. The usual daily dose is 11 milligrams for men and 8 for women.

- *Manganese.* This little-talked-about mineral stimulates enzymes that are important for the production of the amino acid proline, a key component of collagen. Proline, as you might recall from Chapters 1 and

2, helps protect blood vessels, improves joint health, and plays a role in heart health. Manganese is found in brown rice, amaranth, hazelnuts, garbanzo beans, macadamia nuts, oats, white beans, black beans, and buckwheat. You don't need a lot of this mineral — just 2.5 milligrams a day for men and slightly less than 2 for women.

- *Glucosamine.* This naturally occurring compound is known as an "aminosaccharide" because it is made from chains of sugars and proteins bound together. It is abundant in the cartilage of your joints, particularly in the fluid around the joints, where it acts as a natural shock absorber and joint lubricant. Indeed, it has earned a well-deserved reputation for its ability to slow the deterioration of joints and ease joint pain. Not only that, it works with collagen to form the connective tissues that make up parts of the digestive tract and immune system. And glucosamine creates cartilage from proteoglycans, proteins that bolster hydration and load-bearing ability in connective tissue.

Glucosamine is one of the top supplements I recommend as part of a natural approach to arthritis treatment. It's also present in bone broth, so it's naturally part of a collagen-building diet. Glucosamine can also be healing for the gut and minimize jaw pain and bone pain. People often ask me if they should take glucosamine or collagen. The reality is, collagen and glucosamine work synergistically, with glucosamine providing necessary joint lubrication while collagen regenerates and restores aging tissue. Studies show that taking 1,500 milligrams of glucosamine daily can be effective for improving joint health. Take it in 500 milligram doses three times a day.

■ *Chondroitin.* This important structural component of cartilage is one of the key substances, along with glucosamine, that allows joints to retain water and withstand pressure—and studies have shown that it can be moderately effective in relieving joint pain on its own. When it's used in conjunction with glucosamine, it provides greater relief. For instance, in the first phase of the most comprehensive long-term study—the Glucosamine/Chondroitin Arthritis Intervention Trial, known as GAIT—researchers found that the combination of the two substances offered significant relief to study participants with moderate to severe knee pain.[21] The combination treatment also seems to help preserve cartilage and decrease random joint pain in people who don't have arthritis; other research has shown it may help in wound healing. As with glucosamine, it seems to bolster tissue that contains collagen— so using the substances together may be especially effective. The most effective dose of chondroitin is 1,200 milligrams daily in three 400 milligram doses.

■ *Hyaluronic acid.* HA, as it is known, has become the darling of the beauty industry—and for good reason. Hyaluronic acid molecules have a unique ability to bind and retain water, making it especially useful for skin care, since skin better retains its youthful dewiness when it has a high water content. In fact, half of the HA in your body is found in your skin. It also helps boost collagen in the skin and joints. HA is also found in the eyes, fluid around joints, skeletal tissues, heart valves, and lungs; in every location, it plays the important role of maintaining tissue hydration and lubrication. As a result, hyaluronic acid is being used in a variety of different ways—as a supplement to increase overall content, as a topical skin serum or moisturizer, and in eye drops. Daily topical application of serums containing 0.1 percent of HA can help support skin hydration, minimize wrinkles, and bolster elasticity.

Just as collagen levels wane as the years tick by, age and sun exposure take a toll on the size and number of HA molecules in the skin. Taking hyaluronic acid supplements can prevent this decline. Indeed, it has the ability to improve skin's texture and appearance and reduce the signs of aging. What most people don't know is it's also good for reducing joint pain. It's also in bone broth—my favorite collagen-boosting food. When taking HA orally, consume about 50 to 80 milligrams once or twice a day.

Now that you understand the basics of collagen, I hope you're beginning to share my enthusiasm for this remarkable—and largely unappreciated—substance. In the coming pages, I'll lay out the simple dietary tweaks that will help you maximize your body's collagen-producing potential and explain the fascinating research that is revealing the ways in which supporting and amplifying your collagen levels can benefit your appearance and your health — and even add years to your life.

CHAPTER 4

How to Get More Collagen in Your Diet—Starting Today

The Easy Four-Part Approach to Replenish Your Internal Fountain of Youth

Back when I worked directly with patients every day, my most rewarding appointments were follow-up visits. They gave me the opportunity to ask patients about how my suggestions were working. Over the course of those years, I saw hundreds of incredible health transformations. My patients were able to reverse chronic health conditions and, in most cases, get off all—or the majority—of their medications. Whether their pain had receded, their hormones had become more balanced, their gut problems had cleared, they felt more energized, or they'd lost weight, it was always deeply satisfying to know that someone had followed my advice—and become healthier as a result.

Now that I have expanded my mission, I'm able to reach millions of people through social media, YouTube videos, my website, and books, which is a blessing. But I rarely get to see patients one-on-one. So I'm always delighted when people who use my products or participate in my health programs take the time to send me feedback about their results. This note from a woman who participated in our Multi Collagen Makeover program reminded me why I love my job and believe so strongly in trying to help people make the best choices they can about their health:

> I have been wanting to let you know that collagen helped me tremendously. I had upwards of $5,000 worth of cryotherapy done one summer for skin issues. My hair was thin and my nails were brittle and neither was growing. I started using collagen in my smoothies daily, and what a huge difference! My skin issues started disappearing and my nails grew longer and got stronger. My hair has been thickening, and I love it! My body actually needed this. Even my joints feel better. I love collagen, and will continue to use it.

Reading her feedback was a wonderful moment of affirmation. It brought me real joy to hear how she has benefited from collagen. Her story is a great example of what *all* of us stand to gain by adding this powerful substance to our daily diets. Because collagen is woven throughout your body and strongly associated with youthful qualities like strength, healing, elasticity, and flexibility, consuming more of it can reverse some of the most common—and most frustrating and debilitating—collagen-depletion symptoms we all experience as we age.

Supporting your collagen levels isn't just about adding collagen to your diet. To truly make the most of this age-defying protein, you also need to protect your body's current collagen from damage and degradation and take steps to promote the formation of new collagen. To that end, I've created the following three-part dietary approach that bolsters collagen from the inside out and the outside in:

- Eat foods rich in collagen and the amino acids that create collagen, like proline, hydroxyproline, and glycine, including bone broth.
- Consume foods that support your body in creating its own collagen and reduce collagen breakdown, including foods and herbs high in vitamin C, zinc, and polyphenols.
- Avoid foods that destroy the quality and quantity of collagen in your body.

What follows is a comprehensive guide to what you should eat (and what you should steer clear of) to make the most of your body's collagen. This simple, holistic, sustainable nutrition strategy will repair, refresh, and rejuvenate your body's tissues so you remain nimble, active, healthy, and pain-free for years to come.

THE BEST SOURCES OF DIETARY COLLAGEN

Job one is to add collagen to your diet, since at this point, in all likelihood, you're getting almost none. It's always advisable to get as many nutrients as you can from whole foods, and the same holds true for collagen. But given our fast-paced, busy lives, it can be tricky to consume whole sources of collagen every day. So you may need to rely on supplements to round out your collagen intake. With that in mind, here are the collagen-rich foods and supplements you should rely on as you follow my collagen diet meal plan (Chapter 12):

■ *Bone broth.* Hands down my favorite source of collagen, this traditional food has been consumed by humans for millennia. This ancient elixir contains a whopping dose of valuable collagen as well as important minerals — calcium, magnesium, phosphorus, silicon, sulfur, and others — that your body can easily absorb. What's more, it also has glucosamine and chondroitin, two substances that protect joint health.

The bone broths with the most nutrition are the ones you make from scratch at home, using the bones, skin, and gristle from organic, free-range chickens; organic, pasture-raised beef, bison, or lamb; or wild-caught fish. When you brew bone broth from a chicken or turkey carcass, you'll get loads of type II collagen, which is indispensable for joint health. When you simmer the bones of beef, lamb, or bison, you'll create a broth that's rich in the most abundant collagen in your body, type I, as well as type III. Together, these two types of collagen strengthen virtually every body part you can think of: your bones, bone marrow, cartilage, skin, joints, hair, nails, muscles, tendons, ligaments, gums, teeth, eyes, and blood vessels. And when you steep fish bones, scales, and fins, you wind up with a particularly healthy broth that contains one of the most absorbable sources of type I collagen.

■ *Chicken and fish skin.* When you eat free-range chicken and wild-caught fish, don't discard the skin! Season it while you're cooking and consume it along with the meat. It's tasty, and it contains high quantities of easy-to-digest collagen.

■ *Organ meats.* Another source of collagen we've largely rejected is organ meats (also known as offal or glandular meats). Liver, for instance, contains glycine and proline, the amino acids that form the backbone of most of our bodies' collagen. It also has an array of B vitamins, vitamin A, selenium, and folate. When it comes from wild venison, lamb, grass-fed beef, or pasture-raised chicken, liver is a true superfood—more nutrient-dense than kale or spinach. Other organ meats are worth adding to your diet as well. Heart has copious amounts of CoQ10, a potent antioxidant that helps prevent damage to cells, including collagen. Kidney is high in vitamin B12, another antioxidant, as well as selenium, a mineral that protects cells from damage. Sweetbreads, made from the thymus and pancreas, are high in vitamin C, which, as you already know, is a necessary component of your body's internal collagen production.

■ *Gelatin.* As I've mentioned, gelatin is a type of protein derived from collagen that is beneficial for forming strong cartilage and connective tissue. It contains glycine, proline, hydroxyproline, glutamic acid, alanine, arginine, aspartic acid, and lysine. Bone broth is rich in gelatin. And you can make your own gelatin by straining off the gelatinous top layer of bone broth and allowing it to firm up in the refrigerator overnight. It keeps for a week in the fridge, and you can use it as a base for desserts, soups, and stews.

■ *Collagen supplements.* While eating whole foods is preferable, it's not always easy to get enough collagen that way. High-quality supplements are an ideal way to fill the gap. A quick stroll through the supplement section of your local health food store, however, is enough to make your head spin. With the range of options, from gelatin to hydrolyzed collagen to collagen peptides, it's hard to know which ones to choose.

Here are the five things you need to keep in mind to make the best choice:

1. *Look for hydrolyzed collagen or collagen peptides.* Although different products might say one or the other, they're essentially the same thing. Both labels mean the product has undergone a process called hydrolyzation, which breaks collagen molecules down into individual collagen peptides that are easier for your body to absorb. In addition to being more bioavailable, hydrolyzed collagen peptides have a lower molecular weight and can dissolve quickly into nearly any liquid, making them incredibly simple to add to your diet. You can throw a scoop or two in your morning coffee or smoothie, or add it to soup or stew.

2. *Opt for products that contain a wide array of collagen types.* Since the most abundant collagen in your body is type I, any collagen supplement you take should contain it. But because it's important to have an amino acid balance, I believe it's best to find a supplement that has types I, II, III, V, and X, which account for most of the collagen in your body. A multi-collagen product featuring bovine collagen, chicken collagen, fish collagen, and eggshell membrane

collagen ensures that you're getting all five types.

3. *Bone broth protein powder and bone broth collagen powder are great options.* While hydrolyzed multi-collagen protein is wonderful for collagen building, bone broth collagen has an added benefit I mentioned above: It contains glucosamine and chondroitin. If you have arthritis or are starting to develop aches and pains in your joints, a bone broth supplement may be a better option.

4. *Make sure the label specifies the type of collagen the product contains.* If the types aren't listed on the label, there's no way to be sure what you're getting.

5. *Check the dose.* Taking 10 to 30 milligrams daily is ideal for most people. You can take more, especially if you are on a collagen-loading program and looking to help improve collagen deficiencies. However, if the label recommends a super-high quantity, I'd be wary.

ADOPT AN ANTI-INFLAMMATORY DIET

It's not just age that takes a toll on the levels of collagen in your body. It's *inflammation*. You've undoubtedly heard that word a lot, but unless you work in the medical field you might not know exactly what it means. Here's a quick explanation: Inflammation is part of the body's natural immune response to injury and infection, so in many ways it's protective. If you fall and cut your knee, for instance, the area will become swollen and tender—signs that the body is healing and repairing the tissue. However, if you eat a diet high in sugar and processed foods, gain too much weight, experience chronic stress, get too much exposure to UV light, smoke, or get too little sleep or exercise, the body can become chronically inflamed—and that's a big problem. Chronic inflammation is linked to all sorts of dangerous conditions, like heart disease, stroke, depression, and autoimmune diseases. It can also degrade your body's collagen, leading to chronic pain, aging skin, and conditions like osteoarthritis.

But research shows that a nutritious diet of whole, organic foods that come straight from nature supports a healthy inflammation response. As a result, it protects your body's collagen levels, and is a necessary, integral factor in the collagen-boosting equation.

Eating a clean diet has an additional collagen-related advantage: brightly colored vegetables and fruits, the cornerstone of an anti-inflammatory diet, are packed with antioxidants, which fight free radical damage. Free radicals are unstable molecules in the body that are created by normal wear and tear as well as exposure to UV rays, toxins in the environment, and even unhealthy food. They harm other molecules in your body by stripping them of electrons.

It's normal to have some free radicals. In fact, a healthy balance between free radicals and antioxidants supports strong physiological function. But if levels get too high, these rogue molecules can overcome your body's ability to regulate them. This leads to a condition known as oxidative stress, which causes inflammation, accelerates aging, damages cells, and overloads the immune system. Even more concerning, there's evidence that excess free radicals may target proteins in particular — including collagen.

Here's the good news: Research shows that consuming a diet high in antioxidants can keep free radicals in check and protect collagen. A study in the *British Journal of Dermatology,* for instance, found that tomato paste, which is rich in the antioxidant lycopene, can safeguard the collagen in your skin by doing away with free radicals created by sun damage.[22] Other research has shown that consumption of vitamin E, beta-carotene (the red-orange pigment found in carrots and other vibrant veggies), vitamin C, and selenium produces similar protective effects. Likewise, a study in animals in the journal *Atherosclerosis* discovered that antioxidants increase the collagen content inside arteries.[23]

An anti-inflammatory diet has one more important benefit: It includes a variety of healthy foods that contain vitamin C and many of the other collagen cofactors

I talked about in Chapter 3 — substances that bolster your body's ability to absorb and utilize the collagen you get in your diet. If you're interested in doing everything you can to preserve and promote your important collagenous tissue, the very best approach is to augment your diet with indispensable collagen-boosting foods, herbs, and spices that protect your cartilage, skin, tendons, and ligaments from the ravages of age. Fortunately, many of the same foods that fight inflammation are also collagen cofactors.

Here are the anti-inflammatory and antioxidant foods and herbs you should eat regularly to maintain — and fully maximize — your collagen levels:

- *Vegetables.* Dark, leafy greens, like kale, spinach, bok choy, Swiss chard, and collard greens, are great sources of vitamins C, E, and A, plus other collagen cofactors, like zinc, manganese, and copper — all of which support collagen production. They also contain chlorophyll, which increases skin levels of procollagen, a vital component of collagen production. And on top of that, they are excellent sources of antioxidant vitamins and minerals, which reduce inflammation. Bok choy alone contains more than seventy. In addition, both collard greens and spinach contain glutathione, the molecule that has been called the body's master antioxidant because it is the most abundant and active antioxidant in our biological arsenal. The bonus: Glutathione also affects enzymes that protect collagen from degrading. (If you struggle to eat adequate portions of leafy greens, try our delicious anti-inflammatory juice suggestions in Chapters 11 and 12.)

Broccoli, brussels sprouts, cabbage, celery, beets, asparagus, and cauliflower are valuable collagen-protecting allies as well. Asparagus, broccoli, brussels sprouts, and cabbage are super effective at boosting glutathione levels, for instance. And when you eat these wonder foods, your body produces sulforaphane, a substance that has the ability to reduce oxidative stress from free radicals and protect tissues and cells from damage. Similarly, recent pharmacological studies have shown that celery and celery seeds can lower inflammation. Other inflammation-lowering veggies include carrots, butternut squash, sweet potatoes, onions, tomatoes, bell peppers, and eggplant.

And don't forget allium vegetables like garlic, onions, leeks, chives, and shallots. These veggies add tons of flavor to food and pack whopping health benefits, since they're high in flavonols and organosulfur compounds, which make them effective antioxidants and anti-inflammatories. Not only that, sulfur is an essential micronutrient and a critical ingredient for building collagen. Use a quarter cup or so of these flavor boosters in every dish you possibly can, from soups and stews to omelets, pizza, and pasta.

For other fresh vegetables, aim for three to five servings a day. Each serving is about a cup. Half a cup of starchy veggies, like sweet potatoes and squash, is enough.

▪ *Fruit.* Among the most effective anti-inflammatory polyphenols (plant-based nutrients with antioxidant activity) are compounds known as anthocyanins, which give blueberries, strawberries, raspberries, and blackberries their lovely red, blue, and purple hues. One study found that after eating 375 grams of blueberries, people had lower levels of oxidative stress markers and higher levels of anti-inflammatory cytokines in their blood.[24] I'm also a big fan of elderberries, cranberries, acai, maqui, and goji berries, all of which have sky-high ORAC (oxygen radical absorption capacity) scores, which means they're especially good at absorbing and eliminating free radicals. Case in point: One study found that mice, after drinking 5 percent goji juice, had higher levels of protective antioxidants in their skin—and significantly less inflammatory swelling—after sun exposure.[25]

Cherries, grapes, avocados, olives, kiwi, apples, pineapple, oranges, and other citrus fruits all lower inflammation and fight free radicals as well. For instance, a recent literature review published in the *Journal of Oral and Maxillofacial Surgery* found that bromelain, a substance in pineapples, is effective at reducing facial swelling (a type of localized inflammation) in people who've undergone surgery for impacted molars.

Consume one to three servings of fresh fruits daily (a serving is about half a cup).

■ *Fermented foods.* Having a robust population of good bacteria in your gut is critical for reining in inflammation. Here's one key reason why: When you have a preponderance of unhealthy bacteria in your gut, your gut lining becomes more permeable, allowing undigested protein molecules and pathogens into your circulatory system. This triggers your immune system and leads to chronic inflammation. (My book *Eat Dirt* goes into detail about this condition, known as leaky gut.) As a result, it's important to eat foods that support the growth of healthy bacteria, like colorful plant-based foods — as well as fermented foods, the all-stars of the probiotic world.

Fermentation is an age-old preservative process. Our ancestors, who didn't have refrigerators, relied on fermented vegetables, like kimchi, sauerkraut, real pickles (made from scratch, since store-bought pickles usually aren't fermented), and fermented soybeans, like miso, tempeh, and natto, as a key part of their diets. What we now know: When plants' natural sugars become fermented, their probiotic lactic acid bacteria content soars, turning these simple foods into powerful probiotics — and, as a result, super inflammation fighters.

Other fermented foods to add to your diet: grass-fed, organic, unsweetened yogurt; kefir (made from cow, goat, or sheep's milk); and kombucha (made from black tea and sugar). Likewise, raw, organic apple cider vinegar, made from fermented apples, has been used in healing for centuries and can promote gut health; it also is a great source of vitamin C, a terrific collagen booster. Use 1 to 2 tablespoons per day. If you're new to fermented veggies and other foods, start with a half a cup a day and build up gradually to one to two cups a day. This gives your gut time to adjust to the presence of new bacteria. And be sure to eat a variety of fermented foods, since each one contains different beneficial bacteria.

- *Protein.* As I explained in Chapter 2, your body is meant to have a balance of amino acids. So in addition to consuming the amino acids found in collagen, it's also important to get a healthy quantity of other amino acids — many of them *essential* amino acids — from other types of protein. While you should aim to get 25 to 35 percent (or even up to 50 percent if you're over fifty-five or sixty) of your protein from collagen, the rest needs to come from the wholesome, organic protein sources below. If possible, have 20 to 30 grams of protein with every meal. If you're vegetarian or vegan, be sure to eat the recommended daily amount of seeds and nuts, which are good alternative sources.

Wild-caught fish is at the top of my list, because it has a full complement of amino acids, plus it is rich in sulfur. Furthermore, fatty fish, particularly wild-caught salmon, is one of the best sources of omega-3 fatty acids available, putting it in the A-plus category in terms of its ability to slash inflammation. Tuna, sardines, and mackerel are all excellent sources of omega-3s as well. Research shows that people who regularly consume these omega-3-rich types of fish are less likely to develop rheumatoid arthritis, an inflammation-related condition, and omega-3 consumption can help reduce joint inflammation and pain in those who already have the illness. A 3-ounce serving of fish provides 19 to 26 grams of protein. (One word of warning: Farmed fish doesn't have the same nutrients as wild-caught, and I recommend that you avoid it. I also don't recommend shellfish, because it is often contaminated.)

I've already told you about the many benefits of bone broth, but here's one more factor in its favor: It is a powerful inflammation fighter. A study published in the journal *Chest* found that sipping chicken broth reduced the number of white blood cells that cause inflammation-related symptoms, like a stuffy nose.[26]

Grass-fed beef, lamb, venison, and other meats (I don't recommend pork or shellfish, because they are often contaminated with toxins) are important because they contain complete proteins, meaning they give you the full gamut of essential amino acids your body can't live without, plus other nonessentials. They're also an important part of a collagen-bolstering diet, because they contain sulfur, a building block of collagen. A 3-ounce serving of any of these meats provides about 25 to 29 grams of protein.

Pasture-raised poultry, like chicken or turkey, has an amino-acid profile similar to that found in your body. A 3-ounce serving provides 21 to 24 grams of protein. And pasture-raised eggs are rich in a range of amino acids as well as sulfur. Each egg contains about 6 grams of protein.

Meanwhile, raw, organic, and fermented dairy products, like milk, yogurt, kefir, and cheese, offer the complete gamut of essential amino acids, plus calcium and, in the case of yogurt and kefir, gut-healing microbes. One cup of full-fat yogurt, for instance, provides about 8 to 9 grams of protein. I don't recommend any dairy that is processed, because it can be hard on the digestive system.

Plants have protein, too. Legumes, beans, nuts, seeds, 100 percent whole grains, and even some veggies, like leafy greens and cruciferous vegetables, provide a variety of amino acids. But it's important to know that plant proteins are considered incomplete proteins, because they lack one or more of the essential amino acids your body needs. So if you're vegan or vegetarian, be sure to eat a range of plant protein to ensure you're getting all the amino acids you need.

That said, plant protein has a lot going for it. Nuts and seeds are great inflammation fighters, since they contain high levels of inflammation-curbing magnesium, l-arginine, and vitamin E. Walnuts, flaxseed, and chia seeds contain alpha linoleic acid, a type of omega-3 fatty acid — and omega-3s are one of the most potent anti-inflammatories found in nature. Walnuts also contain ellagitannins, a type of polyphenol that your gut converts into a compound that protects the body against runaway inflammation. At the same time, eating a healthy quantity of almonds has been shown to lower some markers of inflammation, including C-reactive protein (CRP).

Moreover, nuts and seeds make healthy, filling snacks and can add crunch and flavor to salads. A half cup of cooked grains, beans, or legumes contains 5 to 9 grams of protein. One cup of vegetables has about 2 to 3 grams.

- *Fats and oils.* Healthy fats, like coconut oil, grass-fed butter, ghee, and organic mayonnaise, should be a part of your daily diet. They support nutrient absorption, appetite control, hormone production, and mental health. Likewise, certain other fats are known for their ability to suppress inflammation. Take extra virgin olive oil (EVOO). High in monounsaturated fats, it also contains polyphenols, like lignans and oleocanthal, which have been associated with lower joint damage in rheumatoid arthritis. Walnut oil is high in alpha-linoleic acid, which, as I mentioned above, can lower levels of C-reactive protein, a key marker of inflammation. Avocado oil, according to studies, seems to lower CRP as well. When purchasing fats and oils, choose organic products whenever possible. And use coconut oil or butter for cooking and EVOO for salad dressing, drizzled over cooked veggies, or as an ingredient in dips and spreads.

- *Herbs and spices.* Even though herbs and spices have been used in healing for eons, in the West they've largely been viewed merely as an easy way to add flavor to food—until now. New studies are shining a light on the health benefits of many everyday herbs and spices, and that research has revealed their ability to tackle out-of-control inflammation and neutralize free radicals. In fact, gram for gram, these flavorful beauties offer more antioxidant protection than vegetables and fruit.

The herbs and spices that should be a part of your collagen-boosting, anti-inflammatory diet include: turmeric, ginger, clove, cinnamon, rosemary, parsley, thyme, sage, oregano, cayenne, black pepper, basil, and mint. They all contain flavonoids that are involved in antioxidant defenses, a healthy inflammation response, and cell renewal. Turmeric, for instance, contains curcumin, a yellow pigment that has strong antioxidant and anti-inflammatory properties, probably because it inhibits certain enzymes that drive inflammation. Ginger contains a variety of anti-inflammatory compounds, including gingerol, shogaol, paradol, and zingerone. A study published in the *Journal of Agricultural and Food Chemistry* found that clove and cinnamon stick are the most potent antioxidants out of the twenty-six herbs and spices studied.[27] Studies of rosemary have repeatedly shown it has anti-inflammatory capacity. Furthermore, research published in *Food and Function* shows that rosemary can reduce inflammation and oxidative stress in rats with arthritis.[28] Get in the habit of using these wonder ingredients liberally when you cook (they're great as a replacement for sugar and salt) and adding them to your bone broth. You can also get creative by making herbal infusions and delicious, delicately flavored teas.

■ *Tonic herbs and mushrooms.* Supplemental herbs and mushrooms can bolster your efforts at minimizing inflammation. For instance, ashwagandha. It's an adaptogenic herb, meaning that its use can help to rectify imbalances in the body, regulating your hormonal response to stress as well as reducing the effects of free radical damage. A study published in the *Journal of Complementary and Integrative Medicine* showed that ashwagandha exhibited antioxidant activity and lowered inflammation in rats with arthritis — effects comparable to those of methotrexate, a commonly prescribed pharmaceutical.[29]

Other adaptogenic herbs used in ancient health care systems like Ayurveda and Traditional Chinese Medicine include Asian and American ginseng, astragalus, and rhodiola. Similarly, a variety of mushrooms possess antioxidant properties, and studies show they may offer protection against collagen degradation and promote collagen synthesis, especially in wound healing. For instance, *Sparassis crispa,* or cauliflower mushrooms, improved wound healing in diabetic rats by promoting the synthesis of type I collagen.[30] Other free-radical-scavenging mushrooms include the extremely common white mushroom, *Agaricus bisporus* (when mature it's known as a portobello); reishi; white oyster mushroom;

and the giant funnel mushroom, whose white cap can grow up to sixteen inches.

■ *Beverages.* The medical field has long recognized that green tea's high antioxidant content offers protection from heart problems and cancer. More recent studies have shown that it has anti-inflammatory properties as well.

I'm a fan of matcha, a high-grade, finely ground concentrated green tea. The leaves are essentially ground up, so instead of discarding the leaves after steeping, as you do when you drink traditional tea, you consume a dissolvable version of the actual leaves. As a result, matcha offers a more potent blend of nutrients and antioxidants called polyphenols, which have an anti-inflammatory effect. I drink a cup or two every day.

Another beverage with anti-inflammatory properties is red wine. It contains resveratrol, a plant-based polyphenol molecule that has been shown to protect cartilage. One study in the *Journal of Medicinal Food* found that high doses of a resveratrol supplement reduced pain and markers of inflammation in those with knee osteoarthritis.[31]

■ *Dark chocolate and cacao nibs.* Who doesn't love chocolate? The good news is that, in moderation, dark chocolate and cacao can be part of a healthy anti-inflammatory diet. Dark chocolate contains flavonoids and polyphenols, both of which fight free radicals. In fact, the content of these substances is higher in dark chocolate's cocoa than in tea or red wine. Look for chocolate that is 70 percent cocoa or higher. Such varieties contain more antioxidants and less sugar. Dark chocolate also contains collagen cofactors, like zinc and manganese. Cacao, which comes from the seeds of fruits of the cacao tree (from which dark chocolate is made), is a superfood in its own right, containing a variety of unique collagen-boosting phytonutrients, including high amounts of sulfur and magnesium. Cacao nibs have more antioxidant activity than tea, wine, blueberries, and even goji berries. Have a few small pieces a day.

AVOID THESE DIETARY COLLAGEN BUSTERS!

Just as there are foods that can protect and enhance your collagen levels, there are ones that can tear it down. In order to preserve this precious tissue, avoid these collagen-destroying foods:

- *Refined carbs.* Crackers, cookies, cereal, pasta, bread, and baked goods contain sugar and chemicals that are damaging to collagen molecules, thereby diminishing the quality of the tissue, and can erode the *quantity* of your collagen as well.
- *French fries and other fried foods.* Fried foods fuel inflammation, creating an internal environment that puts collagen at risk.

■ *Soda and other sugar-sweetened beverages.* Sugar is collagen's nemesis. It causes your insulin to spike, which leads to inflammation. And, as I've mentioned before, it creates advanced glycation end products, also known as glycotoxins, which fuel free radical damage and inflammation.

■ *Processed meats.* Hot dogs, pepperoni, salami, and lunch meats are packed with nitrates and other chemicals that can lead to inflammation. Avoid them if you can.

Knowing what to eat is empowering because it provides you with the basic information you need to choose foods with confidence. The best part: A diet that's healthy for collagen is super nutritious for the rest of your body as well. Reducing inflammation can help you fight almost every other major disease that afflicts Americans today, from heart disease to cancer. So by adopting a collagen-boosting diet you're really committing to a wellness-boosting diet—one that will make you feel and look your best. Here's to enhancing collagen—and your life!

CHAPTER 5

The Six Habits That Supercharge (or Sabotage) Collagen

How to Tweak Your Lifestyle to Protect Your Joints, Skin, and More

We all know that our lifestyle choices have an impact on our health. Even so, in the midst of hectic day-to-day demands, it's super easy to lose sight of our long-term health goals. I'm as guilty as anyone else. When I'm under stress at work, I sleep too little, skip exercise, and become less diligent about my diet. Our bodies are designed to be resilient, so they have the ability to adjust to those challenges in the short term. But if poor habits become the norm—if you're chronically sleep-deprived or sedentary or living on fast food—every system and tissue in your body will suffer, including your collagen.

In previous chapters, we've seen how the modern Western diet leads to collagen deficiency, and how replacing it with an anti-inflammatory diet of whole, organic foods—including lots of antioxidant-rich, collagen-boosting veggies and collagen-rich foods like bone broth and organ meats—can help you shore up your supply of this vital, healthful substance. But it's not just poor nutrition that is taking a toll on collagen; our high-stress lifestyles are also a big problem. In order to keep up with our always-on, hard-driving culture, many of us make daily choices that place undue pressure and stress on this at-risk tissue. So my collagen diet plan isn't just about tweaking your daily eating habits. It's about looking at your whole lifestyle and making small changes that work synergistically with your nutrition-related efforts to have a surprisingly big impact on collagen. By pairing diet with lifestyle, you can support and enhance this turn-back-the-clock tissue and keep yourself feeling and looking young for years to come.

Here are the six healthy lifestyle choices that will safeguard and stimulate collagen—and help you get the most out of the collagen diet. (The bonus: They'll improve your health *and* your state of mind.)

■ *Sit less, move more.* When the American College of Sports Medicine and the American Medical Association officially endorsed the widespread health benefits of movement with their 2007 Exercise Is Medicine initiative, they were echoing an idea that has been promoted by physicians since before Hippocrates. According to ancient records, Susruta, an Indian physician, was the first to recommend exercise to his patients in 600 BCE. "Diseases fly from the presence of a person habituated to regular physical activity," according to Susruta.

He was right, of course, and heeding that ancient wisdom is more vital now than ever. Although the percentage of U.S. adults who meet the weekly exercise recommendations (150 minutes per week of moderate exercise or 75 minutes per week of vigorous aerobic exercise) has risen from about 42 to 53 since 2007, there are still millions of people who are dangerously sedentary. And when it comes to collagen, lack of physical activity can be ruinous. Research shows that those who spend more time sitting have higher levels of C-reactive protein (CRP), an important marker of inflammation. And, as you know from Chapter 4, inflammation attacks collagen, eroding both its volume and its functionality.

That can be quite serious. In addition to the well-known problems associated with collagen deterioration, like skin wrinkling and joint pain, losing this vital tissue can heighten your risk for cardiovascular disease. Studies show that when the collagen in the lining of your arteries wanes with age, your arteries begin to harden, which is an important risk factor for heart disease and high blood pressure.

But here's the good news: Study after study has shown that exercise can reduce inflammation. A recent study published in *Brain, Behavior, and Immunity,* for instance, found that just twenty minutes of brisk walking is enough to trigger an anti-inflammatory response.[32] And a recent literature review in the *European Journal of Clinical Investigation* explained, at least in part, why: When you start moving, your muscle cells release interleukin-6 (IL-6), a protein that lowers levels of compounds that fuel inflammation.[33]

At the same time, research has revealed that moderate-intensity exercise can help build collagen. An animal study published in *Experimental and Therapeutic Medicine,* for instance, found that eight weeks of moderate-intensity running not only increased collagen synthesis in the Achilles tendon but also promoted the quality of the tissue.[34] And another animal study found that both low- and moderate-intensity running significantly increased cartilage thickness in the knee.[35]

If you already exercise, fantastic. Keep it up! If not, now is the time to start. It can be challenging to start a new fitness routine, much less commit to one long term. But here's something to try: Since motivation is notoriously fickle, take it out of the equation as much as possible. Set up a standing walking date with a reliable friend to keep you accountable. Lay out your exercise clothes the night before, so they're the first thing you see in the morning. Find a gym that's near your home or work, so it's easy to get to. When you feel your desire to get out the door waffling, remind yourself of the things you value—good health (including healthy collagen!), increased vitality, the ability to travel or play with your kids—that exercise can deliver.

Don't let tiny slipups derail you; if you miss a day or two because of family obligations or the flu, just chalk it up to life and go back to your routine. And believe in yourself! Research shows that people who believe they have unlimited supplies of willpower seem to exhibit more stick-to-itiveness, not because they're built differently from the rest of us but simply because they believe they can.

■ *Create calm.* Stress in itself isn't a bad thing. Indeed, it's meant to *protect* us. When you're crossing the street and see a car coming at you, or your toddler who can't swim jumps into the pool, it sets off an alarm in the brain, which floods the body with a cascade of hormones that prepare you to fight or flee. Your pulse quickens, your muscles tense, your senses heighten. From time immemorial, this response has protected us from incoming threats, be it a saber-tooth tiger or an oncoming bus. But when stress continues day after day—when you're worried about where your next paycheck is coming from, or going through a divorce, or struggling with a chronic health issue, or on call 24/7 with aging parents—your body stays in that state of high alert and begins to release pro-inflammatory cytokines. And by now you understand why that's dangerous: Inflammation can damage collagen.

There are many ways to tame stress: exercise; reading; taking an Epsom salt bath (the magnesium calms your nervous system); prayer; using essential oils like jasmine, sandalwood, vetiver, and lavender; and taking supplements like ginseng, ashwagandha, rhodiola, and magnesium.

But one of the most effective long-term solutions for coping with stress is mindfulness meditation. It not only helps relax you but also helps you become less reactive to emotional situations. That's important, because better cognitive control is associated with less pronounced pro-inflammatory cytokine reactivity to stress. In a recent study in the journal *Stress,* researchers tested participants to assess their level of cognitive control of emotional information and the levels of pro-inflammatory cytokines in their saliva. Then study subjects viewed either an emotionally evocative video or a neutral video. When the researchers remeasured participants' salivary cytokine levels, they discovered that those who had tested high on cognitive control had significantly lower levels of the inflammation-promoting chemicals after viewing the emotional video.[36] Mindfulness seems to increase cognitive emotional control by building brain areas associated with the skill, like the prefrontal cortex, and by diminishing the size of the amygdala, which is associated with fear and worry.

At the same time, the practice in itself reduces inflammation. In a recent study, researchers from Carnegie Mellon University recruited thirty-five people looking for work—an understandably stressed-out group. Half participated in a three-day mindfulness retreat while the other half did a relaxation retreat. The researchers compared participants' brain scans and blood tests from before the interventions and after. They found that the mindfulness training (but not the relaxation) had rewired participants' brains, creating greater connectivity between two areas: the default mode network, which is active when your mind is wandering, and the executive attention network, which is involved in paying attention and planning. Those who attended the mindfulness retreat also had lower levels of interleukin-6, a key marker of inflammation.[37]

In a similarly intriguing finding, other research has shown that meditation can tame an inflammation-related signaling pathway known as NF-kB, which is associated with aging tissue, including aging skin.[38] In other words, it may play a role in protecting collagen itself.

Mindfulness has been described as "paying attention on purpose." And while it's not necessarily easy, the idea really is that simple. Just sit quietly, close your eyes, and bring your attention to your breathing, the sounds in your environment, or the sensations in your body. Your mind will wander and you'll get distracted.

That's completely normal, so don't let it discourage you. When it happens, simply acknowledge in a non-judgmental way that your mind has strayed, and bring your attention back to your breath (or the sounds or sensations to attend to). Try to do this practice every day for five to ten minutes, and work your way up to twenty to thirty minutes. That small amount is enough to make significant changes in your brain and your ability to cope with everyday challenges.

■ *Embrace sleep.* Get your beauty sleep. How many times have you heard that phrase? Turns out, the advice is solid—and sleep's effect on skin is real. For one thing, the body undergoes necessary repairs during those hours of shut-eye. Studies have shown, for instance, that bone remodeling is interrupted in people who undergo a few days of sleep deprivation. The same thing happens with your skin. While you're asleep, your body releases a variety of chemicals designed to rebuild and repair skin—and a critical part of the rejuvenation process is producing more collagen. And, of course, sleep deprivation is a stress in itself, which means it promotes inflammation.

To take full advantage of the collagen-promoting benefits of sleep, make sure your bedroom is dark and quiet (wear earplugs or use a white noise machine if you're particularly sensitive to noise); keep the temperature at 60 to 67 degrees, the range that is considered optimal for sleep; and set aside eight solid hours on most nights. It can be hard in our go-go-go culture to turn off the TV and computer and crawl into bed. But giving yourself the gift of regular rest can protect your whole body from the ravages of age.

■ *Watch your weight.* On a practical level, carrying too much weight can compress collagen-rich tissues, like knee and spine cartilage, causing them to wear down more quickly than they should. But excess fatty tissue is also dangerous because it, too, can promote inflammation, especially if your weight collects in a spare tire around your belly.

Fat cells release hormones, and research shows that the deep fat that surrounds the organs in your belly, known as visceral fat, is particularly active. They churn out pro-inflammatory cytokines, which helps explain why people who are apple-shaped as opposed to pear-shaped are more likely to develop inflammation-related diseases, like insulin resistance, high blood pressure, type 2 diabetes, and atherosclerosis. As you know, those chemicals also damage collagen.

The best way to get rid of visceral belly fat is through a low-carb, low-sugar diet. The anti-inflammatory diet I lay out in this book is great for weight loss. Another option is the ketogenic diet, which radically reduces carb intake and is worth considering if you have a lot of excess belly fat. (My *Keto Diet* book offers a comprehensive, effective plan for slashing carbs and reducing belly fat.) Other science-vetted strategies include getting daily aerobic exercise; eating more soluble fiber and protein (including collagen protein!), both of which help you feel full longer; and getting plenty of sleep.

■ *Take good care of your mouth.* Gum disease is a notorious driver of inflammation and is a serious risk factor for cardiovascular disease. But simply brushing, flossing, and seeing a dentist regularly for cleanings and check-ups can go a long way toward protecting the health of your gums — as can rinsing your mouth with salt water regularly. A saltwater rinse can kill bacteria and get rid of stray bits of food stuck in your teeth. It can also speed healing of your gums. Just mix a half teaspoon of salt into a glass of warm water and swish around your mouth for thirty seconds several times a day. Practicing good oral hygiene is an often-overlooked way to protect your collagen — as well as your overall health.

■ *Don't smoke.* Take one look at a longtime smoker's skin and you can see for yourself what it does to collagen. But it doesn't just affect the visible collagen in your tissue. In a study reported in *Annals of the Rheumatic Diseases,* researchers followed current smokers and non-smokers, all of whom had osteoarthritis, for thirty months. By the end of the study, they discovered that smokers were more than twice as likely to have significant cartilage loss in their joints as nonsmokers — and smokers experienced more knee pain.[39]

There are a number of possible explanations. For one thing, the toxins in cigarette smoke create free radicals, so smoking increases oxidative stress that contributes to cartilage loss. Additionally, animal studies have found that chondrocytes—cells that produce collagen—become disordered when the animals are exposed to cigarette smoke. So if you need another reason to stay away from tobacco, add protecting your precious supply of collagen to the list.

As you move forward in this book—and as you begin to practice the collagen-promoting plan I've laid out—I'd like you to start working toward embracing a more collagen-friendly lifestyle. Some of you may have a long way to go; others may be almost there. Regardless of where you are on that spectrum, this isn't about perfection. It's about doing what you can and striving for a healthier approach overall. Some of these changes are easier than others, but they'll all pay dividends—and not just when it comes to collagen. Every single one of the strategies I suggest in this chapter will improve your health on a cellular level. They give you more energy, a clearer mind, greater equanimity, and more confidence, which allows you to bring your best self to your family, your friends, your colleagues, and the world.

CHAPTER 6

How Stem Cells Repair and Restore Cartilage and Skin

The New Frontier in Anti-Aging Medicine Is All about Collagen

In the two previous chapters, I've explained dozens of ways you can support your body's natural collagen through diet and lifestyle. Now I'm excited to tell you about a third strategy for regenerating collagen-rich tissue: your body's own stem cells. If you tear a ligament, the new tissue that forms as it slowly knits itself back together comes from stem cells. The same thing happens in your liver. If you have cirrhosis and adopt healthier lifestyle habits, the new organ cells that replace the damaged ones originate from stem cells.

In fact, throughout your life, the stem cells in your bone marrow, body fat, skin, muscles, blood vessels, and brain have been working diligently behind the scenes to patch up and rebuild injured or damaged tissues—including those with the highest collagen content, like your skin, ligaments, tendons, cartilage, spinal disks, gut, and blood vessels.

The stem cells responsible for this remarkable act of regeneration are known as *adult* stem cells. (They're not the controversial embryonic stem cells you've undoubtedly heard about, but I'll explain more about those later.) The human body has more than two hundred types of cells. Each has a specific size, shape, and skill set that makes it perfectly suited to its function in the body. Except stem cells. They're *nonspecific*—in other words, they aren't assigned one particular role. But they have a unique superpower: They're the only cells that can transform into other types of cells—be it tendon, liver, muscle, blood, or brain—and seamlessly integrate into the distinct body parts where those cells belong to revitalize and renew the existing tissue.

As a result, adult stem cells are key players in your body's internal healing system. Sometimes they undertake repairs on their own. For instance, in the skeletal muscle, gut, bone marrow, and brain, adult stem cells continually transform into new specialized cells to replace those that are damaged through injury, illness, or normal wear and tear.

Other times, adult stem cells lie dormant for years, as often happens in the pancreas and heart. Then, when these organs incur damage—from a heart attack, for instance—the body activates these versatile cells, and they move in to mend the organ and replace its worn-out and impaired cells.

And now, thanks to recent medical advances, doctors are increasingly using patients' own stem cells to help them overcome injuries and diseases. From regenerating cartilage, tendons, ligaments, and skin to repairing damaged hearts, fighting cancer, and fending off Alzheimer's, stem cells are beginning to take on greater importance in medicine. As science continues to reveal what these cells are capable of, they will undoubtedly play an ever-larger role in treatments of the future.

While the idea of using stem cells to treat illness is new and exciting, a similar concept, known as *jing,* or essence, has existed in Traditional Chinese Medicine for several thousand years. *Jing* is considered the origin of life. Similarly, embryonic stem cells—those that are present when a recently fertilized egg is three to five days old—give rise to the entire body and every cell in it. *Jing* deficiency is caused by chronic disease, stress, and aging—some of the same hazards that damage and deplete stem cells. And, as I'll explain in more detail below, Chinese herbs meant to nourish *jing* are increasingly being shown to promote stem cell proliferation and differentiation.

Both Eastern and Western medicine agree: Having a healthy population of stem cells ready to swing into action when needed is vital for healthy aging—and healthy collagen. But stem cells age, just like other cells in your body, and they're susceptible to many of the same degrading insults, like poor diet and inflammation. Fortunately, there are steps you can take to protect this internal source of healing.

Let's take a look at how stem cells come to the rescue when collagen-rich tissue is damaged, as well as the simple steps you can take—including the use of Chinese herbs—to help you maintain a thriving population of these remarkable cells, which provide your body with the ability to regenerate collagen and heal itself.

HOW STEM CELLS PROMOTE HEALING

In 2005, Bartolo Colón, a longtime starting pitcher in Major League Baseball, won the American League Cy Young Award, an honor that goes to the league's best pitcher. In the years that followed, he struggled with injuries and was shunted from team to team. Toward the end of the 2009 season, he was sidelined by an elbow injury, and he sat out all of 2010. It looked like that moment in 2005 had been the pinnacle of his quickly diminishing career. Then, suddenly, in 2011 he was back—and throwing ninety-five-mile-per-hour fastballs. He retired in 2019, after twenty-one seasons—at age forty-six.

How did "Big Sexy," as fans called him, manage to play another eight years of Major League Baseball after sustaining injuries that are often career ending? In 2010, doctors harvested stem cells from Colón's own body fat and bone marrow and injected them into the damaged ligaments around his elbow and the torn rotator cuff in his shoulder. The cells worked to repair the damage in Colón's joints, restoring their collagen levels and, as a result, their functionality.

Colón's astonishing, stem-cell-driven comeback was the first to be reported in the media—but he wasn't the first athlete to use the treatment to repair injured tendons, cartilage, or bone tissue. And he definitely wasn't the last.

By now hundreds of pro athletes, as well as high school and college hopefuls, have received stem cell therapy. Before he retired, Alex Rodriguez, who played shortstop and third base, used it to repair an injured knee. Tiger Woods had stem cell treatments to rejuvenate his knee tendons. Kobe Bryant used his body's own platelet rich plasma, which supports stem cells, to help repair a torn Achilles during his NBA comeback. And Super Bowl–winning quarterback Peyton Manning had stem cell injections to heal a neck injury.

You've probably heard a bit about stem cell therapy, the cornerstone of the surging new field of regenerative medicine. But here's something you most likely *don't* know: The approach is an innovative way to surgically renew collagen, because it has the potential to literally turn back the clock on aging collagen-infused tissues, like cartilage, tendons, ligaments, and bones.

That's what seems to have happened with Bartolo

Colón and hundreds of other athletes who've returned to play after stem cell therapy. Colón's doctor used so-called mesenchymal adult stem cells (MSCs) in his treatment. They're found in bone marrow, fat cells, dental tissue, and skin, where they give rise to a variety of different types of specialized cells, like bone, muscle, and fat. But MSCs can also transform into cartilage cells called chondrocytes, which produce the extracellular matrix in which collagen resides; in other words, they're particularly useful for regenerating collagen.

Thanks to their ability to infuse cartilage with new life, MSCs have been shown to be helpful in healing soft-tissue-related injuries and illnesses. For a small study in the *International Journal of Rheumatic Diseases,* for instance, researchers injected MSCs into the joints of patients with severe osteoarthritis and found they reported a significant improvement in pain as well as the number of stairs they could climb; when the researchers followed up with study subjects five years later, the knees that had been treated had deteriorated somewhat, but they still functioned better than they had before the treatment.[40] Likewise, a study in *Transplantation* revealed that injecting MSCs into arthritic joints can improve patients' cartilage quality[41] — which means it improves collagen quality as well.

Researchers believe that stem cells not only help heal tissue directly, by creating new cells, but also create a healing environment that promotes cellular rejuvenation.

Mesenchymal stem cells produce anti-inflammatory cytokines, for instance. They also secrete growth factors, which stimulate cell proliferation and promote the production of the collagen-filled extracellular matrix. At the same time, they signal the body to deliver nutrients and other substances required for cellular repair.

While stem cells are an exciting new tool for helping repair injured connective tissue, their healing promise extends beyond anatomical issues. Bone marrow transplants, which transfer blood stem cells to patients, have been used for more than fifty years to treat blood disorders like leukemia and lymphoma. What's more, studies are under way to determine if stem cell therapy could one day change the course of devastating conditions like Alzheimer's disease, Parkinson's, spinal cord injuries, and even heart disease, cancer, and type 1 diabetes.

As I mentioned earlier, stem cell therapy is often viewed as controversial, largely because of its connection with embryonic stem cells (ESCs). Embryonic stem cells have more versatility than adult stem cells. They can become *any* type of cell, whereas adult stem cells' transformation options are somewhat more limited. However, that versatility has a downside. For example, ESCs may transform into the wrong cell types, causing tumors and other problems. And the immune system sometimes sees ESCs as foreign invaders and attacks the new tissue they form.

The other concerning issue is that ESCs are harvested from early-stage embryos not long after fertilization takes place. The cells are retrieved from in vitro fertilization clinics, which typically have a supply of extra embryos that were not used by patients; in order to use these embryos for stem cell research, doctors need informed consent from the donors. The National Institutes of Health also has guidelines that define how these cells can be used in scientific studies. But understandably, some people object to using embryonic tissue for research.

The field of regenerative medicine is new, and researchers are still discovering how best to grow stem cells in a lab, what conditions they're most effective in treating, and how to utilize them to optimize healing, but I think it's important for you to understand the state of play when it comes to how stem cells heal and restore collagen-rich tissue, as well as their medical potential.

I believe the treatment may one day offer next-level healing for many people who have sustained joint- or bone-related injuries as well as those who want to keep their bodies as young and high-functioning as possible well into old age.

HOW TO SUPPORT YOUR STEM CELLS (SO THEY CAN PROTECT YOUR COLLAGEN!)

As I mentioned earlier, stem cells age, just like all other living organisms. However, the aging of stem cells carries greater significance, according to some researchers. They've formulated the "stem cell theory of aging," which speculates that the human body's aging process is the *result* of aging stem cells. In other words, as stem cells get older and become less capable of replenishing tissues and organs with sufficient numbers of new cells to maintain their function, our bodies themselves show more signs of wear and tear, falling into decline and disrepair.

The theory makes a certain amount of sense. After all, stem cells, more than any other types of cells, are responsible for rejuvenating our tissue. And regardless of whether stem cells are responsible for aging or simply play an active role in the process, we know that these remarkable cells, along with the collagen they create, can help keep our bodies more youthful. As a result, it makes sense to do everything we can to protect this elegant, built-in, biological repair system.

Like collagen—and pretty much every other tissue in your body—stem cells thrive in a wholesome, low-inflammation environment. The dietary guidance I provided in Chapter 4 will go a long way toward creating the ideal internal milieu to foster stem cell replication and differentiation. But here are six other ways you can help your supply of stem cells thrive:

- *Slash your sugar consumption*. That means staying away from sweets *and* limiting simple carbs, which cause a surge in blood sugar that's almost as extreme eating a candy bar. Need motivation? In a study looking at stem cell function in the adipose tissue of people with and without diabetes, researchers at Tulane University Health Science Center found that elevated glucose in both groups (but especially diabetics) reduced stem cells' ability to proliferate and turn into cartilage or bone cells—and could actually cause stem cell death.[42] Limiting sugar, on the other hand, improves adult stem cell function and also prolongs the cells' life span.[43]

■ *Try short-term fasting.* Studies have long shown that fasting can be good for the body. Now, research has revealed that it can give stem cells a boost, too. For instance, biologists from the Massachusetts Institute of Technology recently reported that a twenty-four-hour fast can reverse the age-related loss of intestinal stem cells in mice[44]—a vital finding, since intestinal stem cells are responsible for maintaining the lining of the intestine, which renews every five days, as well as repairing damage from infections or injuries. As you age, the population of stem cells in your gut shrinks, making it more difficult to recover from gastrointestinal infections. Scientists don't understand precisely how fasting helps, but here's what we know so far: When mice go without food for a full day, it triggers a metabolic switch that prompts intestinal stem cells to begin burning fatty acids instead of glucose, and, for reasons that aren't entirely clear, shifting from glucose to fat revives the regenerative capacity of stem cells and significantly enhances their function.

Similarly, another study in mice, reported in the journal *Cell,* found that not eating for even a few hours can elevate muscle stem cell activity—and the approach worked well in both young and old rodents.[45]

■ *Stay strong—and active.* There's lots of research showing that exercise is good for stem cells—and having healthy stem cells is vital for the body's ability to repair muscle tissue, along with cartilage, tendons, ligaments, and bones. Studies have shown that aerobic exercise increases the total number of bone-marrow-derived mesenchymal stem cells and restores muscle stem cell mobilization and regenerative capacity.

In one study, Polish researchers had a group of mice run on a treadmill at progressive speeds over a five-week period. At the end of the training, the researchers compared the quantity of the mesenchymal stem cells in their bone marrow with that of sedentary mice. They found that the fit mice had significantly higher numbers of stems cells than the sedentary group, and those stem cells were primed to create new specialized bone cells. They concluded that exercise may represent a novel, nonpharmacological strategy for slowing the age-related decline of musculoskeletal functions.[46] (Other studies have revealed similar findings for muscle cells.) *And* studies looking at stem cell transplants show that exercise stimulates your chondrocytes to grow new collagen-rich cartilage.

The specific type and intensity of exercise may be less important than the movement itself, seeing as everything from strength training to yoga seems to help, and mild to relatively vigorous exercise has been shown to be effective. If you have trouble motivating yourself to get to the gym or hop on your bike or go for a run, think of your stem cells and collagen—and do it for them.

■ *Get enough sleep.* You already know how important sleep is, but the health of your stem cells is yet another reason to make sure you get adequate rest. Stanford researchers found that hematopoietic stem cells (the type used in stem cell transplants for a variety of malignant and nonmalignant diseases) in sleep-deprived mice showed an alarming decrease in activity. In fact, a sleep deficit of just four hours triggered a 50 percent drop in stem cells' ability to transform into specialized cells in the blood and bone marrow.[47] And chances are, the same forces that damage one type of stem cell take a toll on the others, including those that help maintain healthy collagen. Is that extra episode of your favorite binge-worthy TV show really worth it?

■ *Reduce stress.* Earlier in this chapter, I mentioned Traditional Chinese Medicine's concept of *jing* and how similar it is to the modern practice of using stem cells to treat illness. Here's another correlation: Stress, which takes a substantial toll on *jing,* is also a nemesis of stem cells. Here's one interesting example of what stress can do to stem cells: In a study published in the journal *Cell Death Discovery,* researchers restrained mice with liver injuries as a way to induce psychological stress. In response, the mice secreted corticosterone, a stress hormone, which impaired the ability of the rodents' mesenchymal stem cells to differentiate into the types of cells needed to repair the damaged tissue in the liver.[48]

■ *Add these foods to your diet.* In addition to eating the anti-inflammatory foods I suggest in Chapter 4 — especially bone broth, since the bone marrow it contains is a potent source of mesenchymal stem cells — make sure you get plenty of these stem-cell-boosting beauties in your diet: Vitamin D3, which can reduce the aging of stem cells and bolster their ability to differentiate into other types of cells, for instance, and vitamin C, which can bolster stem cell production.

Likewise, researchers at the Medical College of Georgia found that epigallocatechin-3-gallate (EGCG), a free-radical-killing polyphenol in green tea, accelerates the differentiation of stem cells in human skin and can even encourage older skin cells, which normally would die off, to become more robust and live longer.[49] (Matcha green tea is my favorite because it's actually made from ground-up leaves of the *Camellia sinesis* plant. The leaves aren't dried, as they are with most tea, so matcha contains a higher level of antioxidants and chlorophyll, which is a potent detoxifier that can help your body eliminate damaging chemicals and heavy metals.) And several studies show that goji berry extract can promote mesenchymal stem cells; due to its stem-cell-boosting potential, some companies are even working it into skin care formulas to rejuvenate aging skin.

Spirulina, a type of seaweed found in alkaline lakes in Africa and Central and South America, can be effective, too. One study in mice found that eating spirulina for 28 days produced new neural stem cells and protected existing stem cells from the dangerous effects of inflammation[50]—an effect spirulina likely has on all types of stem cells.

I'm a fan of zinc as well. It's an essential element required for stem cell division, migration, and proliferation, and it has also been found to encourage stem cells to proliferate and transform into other types of specialized cells. Foods rich in zinc include grass-fed lamb and beef, garbanzo beans, cashews, pumpkin seeds, plain whole fat yogurt, chicken, turkey, eggs, mushrooms, and salmon.

■ *And don't forget these TCM herbs and foods for building and protecting* jing *and protecting stem cells.* Schisandra berry helps to balance the *jing* with the two other treasures of the body, the *shen*—our spirit or mind—and the *qi,* our life source or bodily energy.

Eggs and fish roe are often used to build and replenish *jing.* Indeed, eggs are nutritional powerhouses packed with vitamin B12, folate, and vitamin D, and fish roe has antioxidant and anti-aging potential thanks to its high concentration of protein and omega-3 fatty acids.

Reishi is known as the king of mushrooms in TCM. Traditional practitioners dry the mushroom, cut it into slices, and boil it in hot water to make a healing soup or tea that nourishes the heart, preserves liver health, promotes a sense of calm, slows aging, and enhances vitality, strength, and stamina.

Panax ginseng is used in TCM to enhance longevity, among other things, and studies show it promotes the proliferation and differentiation of neural stem cells.

Fo-ti root is a Chinese herbal medicine derived from the *Polygonum multiflorum* plant. Revered in the TCM world for its ability to fight aging—it's often prescribed for premature graying—its benefits are due to its whopping supply of antioxidants. Indeed, research suggests that fo-ti's anti-inflammatory effects are similar in strength to those of prescription anti-inflammatory medications. The primary essence of fo-ti is *jing*.

Astragalus is a plant in the legume family, and studies have shown it has a number of effects on stem cells. A study in *Medical Science Monitor,* for instance, found it can regulate inflammation of mesenchymal stem cells;[51] and a paper in *Biomedicine & Pharmacotherapy* found that astragalus promotes proliferation and differentiation of mesenchymal stem cells in bone marrow, in part by activating an intracellular signaling pathway that plays a role in regulating the cell cycle, including proliferation.[52]

Rehmannia, a type of flowering perennial plant, is considered to be a "general tonic" by both TCM and Japanese medicine, meaning it can help a wide variety of symptoms and health concerns. A study published in *Genetics and Molecular Research* found that after four weeks of treatment with rehmannia, rats' bone marrow mesenchymal stem cells were induced to differentiate into heart muscle cells.[53] What's more, lab research published in *Life Sciences* showed that rehmannia could increase the viability and proliferative capacity of fat-derived mesenchymal stem cells—and it achieved that result by secreting two types of growth factors. Furthermore, when the researchers administered hydrogen peroxide to the cells to kill them, rehmannia prevented many of the cells from dying.[54]

I know you care about anti-aging breakthroughs as much as I do, so I'm delighted to be able to share this information on the importance of stem cells and the vital—and largely unsung role—they play in keeping your collagen healthy and abundant. If we want to shield our connective tissue, joints, gut, organs, and skin from the havoc of age, protecting our stem cells must be part of the strategy.

PART II

What Collagen Can Do for You

CHAPTER 7

Collagen Can Create Luminous Skin, Hair, and Nails

The Ancient Herbs, Superfoods, and Essential Oils That Will Bolster Your Beauty Routine

You peer closely in the mirror one day and notice small crow's-feet at the corners of your eyes and fine lines around your mouth. Your skin isn't as bright as it once was, and it doesn't feel as springy and elastic. Sound familiar? If so, I'm glad you're here. While these signs of aging are perfectly normal (though exacerbated by bad habits, like too much sun exposure, sugar consumption, stress, and smoking), they're typically the first, most visible signal from your body that your collagen is on the wane. And those hallmarks of aging skin gradually become more noticeable as the years tick by, since, as you'll recall, there's evidence that older adults produce up to 75 percent less collagen than those younger than thirty.

Research shows that the most evident and reproducible biological feature of aging skin is the atrophy of the extracellular matrix, which is caused by a decrease in the number of fibroblasts (the cells that produce collagen) and a reduction in the quantity and quality of the collagen and elastin. The majority of those changes are driven by inflammation and free radical damage—which is why, in Chapter 4, I emphasized the importance of eating an anti-inflammatory, antioxidant diet.

But there's good news: No matter your age, you can rein in the typical effects of aging on your skin, hair, and nails by adding collagen to your diet. (Although collagen in skin care products is beneficial, too, consuming collagen is more effective.) Indeed, collagen's ability to preserve and refresh skin, and, to a lesser degree, hair and nails, has been more widely studied than any of its other uses. By now, paper after paper supports its effectiveness.

■ A number of studies, including papers published in the journals *Skin Pharmacology and Physiology*,[55] *Nutrients*,[56] and the *Journal of the Science of Food and Agriculture*,[57] have found that using collagen supplements for four to twelve weeks improves skin hydration, elasticity, and wrinkles—the preeminent signs of aging skin, and the top skin-related concerns of most people who want to improve their appearance. What's more, the trials revealed that older people respond as robustly to the supplements as younger subjects—sometimes more robustly. These papers reveal that collagen is able to reduce crow's-feet and other wrinkles by stimulating procollagen 1, a collagen precursor, along with other aspects of the body's collagen-making machinery. For instance, collagen ingestion leads to an increase in the number of collagen-making fibroblasts in the skin, so it effectively revs up the engine that is responsible for producing both collagen and elastin, the substance that allows skin to resume its shape after being poked, pinched, or stretched, giving skin a multi-level youth boost.

▪ In a double-blind, randomized, placebo-controlled trial published in *Nutrition Research*, sixty participants consumed a hydrolyzed fish collagen supplement that also contained vitamins, antioxidants, chondroitin, and glucosamine, while sixty others consumed a sham product. After ninety days, those who were given the collagen-based supplement had significantly more elasticity in their skin than those in the control group, and biopsies showed an improvement in the organization of their skin's collagen fibers, which is important, since one of the red flags of aging is a fragmentation of the skin's collagen network.[58] The study in the *Journal of Cosmetic Dermatology* that I mentioned in Chapter 3 also found reduced collagen fragmentation in the skin to be associated with collagen supplementation.

This indicates that one of the most important effects of ingestible collagen is that it can bolster the *quality* of the collagen in your skin, thereby improving its ability to keep the tissue taut, pliable, and elastic.

■ In a randomized, controlled trial published in the *Journal of Medicinal Food,* researchers recruited 105 women with moderate cellulite. Some of the participants were given a daily 2.5-gram collagen supplement, while others received a placebo. After six months, those who had been taking the collagen supplement had a noticeable improvement in the appearance of their cellulite compared to those who were given the sham treatment. The effect was more pronounced in women who were a normal weight than in those who were overweight, but both groups experienced improvement, leading the researchers to summarize their findings this way: "Based on the current data, it can be concluded that long-term therapy with orally administered bioactive collagen peptides leads to an improvement of cellulite and has a positive effect on skin health."[59]

■ And a small double-blind placebo-controlled study published in the journal *Marine Drugs* looked at people who drank a supplement containing fish collagen combined with ornithine, a nonprotein amino acid that has been shown in some studies to increase levels of hormones that have a beneficial effect on the skin. By the end of the eight-week trial, those in the supplement group had significantly more elastic and well-hydrated skin; they also had higher plasma levels of insulin-like growth factor-1, a substance that contributes to skin development and maintenance and correlates with growth hormone—a key driver of skin cell growth, proliferation, and regeneration. In other words, adding collagen and ornithine to the diet activated the machinery underlying youthful cell turnover and glowing skin.[60]

Given the results of these studies, it's safe to say that collagen can stand up to the most effective skin care products on the market. And in addition to the impressive—and growing—body of science showing that collagen works, people who use it rave about its effects on their skin. Although testimonials are no substitute for science, they're valuable in their own right; like user reviews on Amazon or Rotten Tomatoes, they offer an unvarnished glimpse of the opinions and experiences of real people in the real world.

With that in mind, here is some of the feedback I've received from people who participated in my Multi Collagen Makeover program:

Jeanelle said: "My skin is much brighter after consuming collagen every day for the past three weeks. The results are undeniable. And I love that I can mix it into any beverage without a bitter aftertaste."

Betty said: "Before taking collagen, my hair was falling out. Now it's coming back in thick. I'm very satisfied, and I want to thank you!"

A woman who didn't provide her name said: "I will be sixty at the end of the year. I was looking for something to address issues with my skin and hair. Hair is starting to fall out more than I like. Facial skin losing elasticity. Neck is getting major wrinkles and getting crepey. Just one week after taking collagen I started noticing some changes. Now crepey neck is gone. Face and neck are getting smoother and tighter. For me, this product works wonders."

None of this feedback should come as any surprise — especially when you understand what collagen does in the skin. Up to 80 percent of the skin's protein is collagen — and protein is the stuff that acts as a support network for the dermis, the layer that helps keep the tissue resilient and supple. That vital support structure is pivotal for preventing wrinkles and dry, dull skin.

Your hair and nails need collagen, too. Hair is primarily made of the protein keratin, and keratin construction relies on proline, one of the main amino acids in collagen. Not only that, research shows that hair thinning and loss, a common problem associated with aging, is caused in part by hair follicle shrinkage, which can be the result of free radical damage; and, as you already know, collagen, especially from fish, is a potent antioxidant. Even more intriguing, one study in *Science* linked hair follicle health with type XVII collagen.[61]

Although the link between collagen and overall hair quality has been the subject of very little scientific research, I've heard plenty of stories from women who have taken collagen and rave about its effects on their hair. And a study in the *Journal of Drugs in Dermatology* looking at a proprietary substance that contains collagen as well as other anti-inflammatory and anti-oxidant ingredients found that women with thinning hair experienced a significant improvement in hair growth, volume, and thickness after using the supplement for six months—and, according to a macrophotography analysis, there was a statistically significant increase in the number of new immature hair strands after just three months.[62]

Research on nails is somewhat scarce as well, but a study in the *Journal of Cosmetic Dermatology* found that participants who consumed 2.5 grams of a collagen supplement once a day for twenty-four weeks had a 12 percent increase in the rate of their nail growth and a 42 percent decrease in broken nails, a sign of brittleness.[63] At the end of the trial, 80 percent of participants said they were happy with the results—a finding that echoes reports I've heard from patients, friends, and family, including my sister, who have used collagen over the years.

Clearly, collagen can have an impact on your appearance. But here's the thing: It doesn't operate in a vacuum. In fact, it works best when it's used in conjunction with a variety of other strategies that support and promote its production. In the coming pages, I'll provide a quick overview of microneedling and red light therapy, which can increase collagen in the skin, then move on to other ways to support skin collagen. From herbs and spices to essential oils and superfoods—dozens of collagen-boosting substances are *also* great for your skin, hair, and nails.

THE THREE BEAUTY TREATMENTS THAT CAN ENHANCE YOUR SKIN'S COLLAGEN

There are dozens of beauty treatments on the market, many of which can improve your skin's appearance. But because I know how important collagen is for turning around aging skin, these three approaches are my favorites—and are worth a try.

■ *Red light therapy.* Light therapy is actually an ancient healing tradition, with roots in the medical traditions of Egypt, Greece, China, and India. In this contemporary version, low-power, red light waves are shined on the skin. Red light can be absorbed by the skin to a depth of about eight to ten millimeters, allowing it to penetrate into the dermis, the skin layer where most of your collagen resides. Studies have shown that light in the spectral range of 600 to 1,300 nanometers—red light is 620 to 700 nanometers—is useful for promoting wound healing, tissue repair, and skin rejuvenation. (By the way, red light doesn't have the more dangerous UVA or UVB rays that have been linked to skin cancer and premature aging.) It pulls off this magic trick by stimulating cell proliferation. Specifically, red light therapy regenerates fibroblasts, the cells that give rise to collagen.

A study published in *Photomedicine and Laser Surgery* found that participants treated with red light therapy had reduced wrinkles and fine lines, as well as improved skin tone and increased collagen density confirmed through ultrasonographic measurements.[64] At the same time, the therapy has been shown to be moderately effective for reversing hair loss and stimulating follicle growth. A literature review of the technique (also known as low-level laser therapy) by researchers from Massachusetts General Hospital and Harvard Medical School concluded that it can stimulate hair growth in both men and women and may work by triggering epidermal stem cells in the hair follicle to shift into production mode.[65]

- *Microneedling.* Also known as collagen induction therapy, microneedling is a minimally invasive skin treatment performed by moving a tool with tiny needles over the skin, making minuscule punctures in the top layer. Although you can do it at home if you have a microneedling tool, it's safest to have the treatment done by an experienced dermatologist or aesthetician. The infinitesimal wounds send the skin into repair mode and trigger the body to ramp up collagen and fibroblast production.

A study published in *Plastic and Reconstructive Surgery* found that patients treated one to four times experienced a notable improvement in wrinkles, scarring, and stretch marks—and they showed a significant increase in collagen and elastin six months after treatment.[66] Likewise, a study published in the *Journal of Cutaneous and Aesthetic Surgery* examined how well the treatment worked in patients with deep acne scars; when the study was over, the majority of participants had measurable decreases in the severity of their scarring, and more than 80 percent rated their treatment as excellent on a ten-point scale.[67]

Microneedling might bolster hair growth, as well. Research in mice has shown enhanced expression of hair-related genes and stimulation of hair growth in mice that underwent microneedling. One study in humans showed that when microneedling was used in conjunction with Minoxidil, a prescription hair loss treatment, it was more effective than Minoxidil alone.[68]

- *Exercise.* Okay, so it's not a beauty treatment per se, but I had to mention working out here, because getting your sweat on, whether through aerobic exercise or strength training, increases the production of growth hormone. And growth hormone, as I've mentioned, prompts your fibroblasts to churn out more collagen. Although most forms of exercise seem to trigger growth hormone, the latest research indicates that strength training and interval training (also known as burst training) are the most effective. And putting the two together may offer the biggest bang for the buck.

In a study published in *PLOS One,* researchers recruited healthy young and middle-aged volunteers to participate in a thirteen-week training program, which alternated between two types of training. During one session, participants did interval training— including three to five sets of running or cycling at maximum velocity followed by passive recovery for two to three minutes. Two days later, they returned for a resistance training session. For the resistance training, participants used progressively heavier weights and did five to six exercises that targeted all the major muscle groups. When compared to a control group, who did not participate in the program, those in the exercise group had significantly higher levels of growth hormone at rest and in response to a sprint exercise. Equally intriguing, before the exercise program, the younger participants' growth hormone levels were higher; after the thirteen-week training program, the age difference with regard to growth hormone had disappeared.[69] This suggests that a combination training program can help those in midlife attain a more youthful level of collagen-boosting hormones.

And don't forget adaptive exercise, like yoga. It, too, can be great for keeping your skin youthful and fresh, because it reduces stress, a collagen killer, and the side-bending and downward poses deliver a healthy dose of healing blood and oxygen to your whole body, including your skin. Moreover, levels of glutathione, the powerful antioxidant I mentioned in Chapter 4, are higher in people who do yoga regularly, while stress hormone levels are lower,[70] making the internal environment of your body more collagen-friendly. I swear by yoga's stress-reducing benefits, and so does my wife, Chelsea. If you're not already a practitioner, I suggest you add it to your usual fitness routine at least one day a week.

THE HERBS AND ESSENTIAL OILS THAT GIVE COLLAGEN AN EXTRA BOOST

The true secret to skin health lies not in what you put onto your skin but in what you put into your body. And collagen is without a doubt the most effective form of edible skin care. But its results can be bolstered by a number of other lifestyle habits. The anti-inflammatory diet from Chapter 4 will supercharge your efforts to consume more collagen. What's more, many ancient herbs and spices, both dried and fresh, along with essential oils (some of which you apply to your skin) and superfoods, have antioxidant and anti-inflammatory effects that help prevent the loss or degradation of collagen and promote radiant skin. I already told you about some of them in Chapter 4. But a number of true powerhouse ingredients are worthy of a quick additional mention here. Once you understand how and why they work, you'll see why I believe you should add them to your routine.

The use of plant extracts and herbs to improve appearance has roots in ancient times, with mentions in medical texts and other writings from ancient China and Egypt. These long-ago practitioners didn't know specifically how the plants worked, but through trial and error and repeated use, they discovered the unique benefits of each shrub, leaf, and flower. Now science is starting to support and explain what the ancients discovered long ago. While herbs' mechanisms of action differ, they seem to protect skin on a cellular level, often triggering fibroblasts, the cells that produce collagen, to swing into action.

Ancient superfoods are similar. They've been used in medicine throughout the ages, and now, with the help of modern scientific methods, we're beginning to appreciate how and why they're so beneficial for skin health. The same goes for essential oils. Derived from plants, they contain concentrated amounts of active compounds that naturally support a healthy inflammation response, one of the many ways they boost skin health. Here's a look at a few of these substances — and why and how they can protect the collagen in your skin.

My three favorite skin-perfecting herbs and spices:
Turmeric. As you already know, one of the primary

drivers of skin aging is free radical damage, and when it comes to battling reactive oxygen species, turmeric is a rock star. That means it's highly likely to do good things for your skin, like prevent moisture loss and protect against wrinkles. At the same time, curcumin, the active ingredient in turmeric, is beneficial for wound healing, possibly because it shortens the inflammatory phase of the process. It also appears to facilitate collagen synthesis as well as fibroblast migration and replication, according to a paper in the *International Journal of Molecular Sciences*.[71]

Cinnamon. Who doesn't love cinnamon? And it turns out this delicious spice's active component, cinnamaldehyde, actually promotes type I collagen synthesis within skin fibroblasts, according to research in the *Journal of Agricultural and Food Chemistry*.[72] Researchers believe it works by triggering insulin-like growth factor-1 signaling, which stimulates growth hormone.

Ginger. Like turmeric, ginger is a powerful antioxidant, so it prevents skin aging at its source by eliminating free radicals. Ginger's impressive antioxidant capacity can also protect collagen, research shows. One study in *Wound Repair and Regeneration* found that when ginger is combined with curcumin, it can promote wound healing—and collagen production[73]—so consider using both in recipes whenever possible.

The four best ancient superfoods for skin support:
Amla berry. According to research in the *Journal of*

Ethnopharmacology, amla berry extract increases mitochondrial activity in the skin's fibroblasts (mitochondria are the energy-generating structures within cells) and promotes the production of procollagen, the precursor to collagen.[74]

Ginseng. This potent, inflammation-reducing antioxidant may help your skin, too. Panax ginseng root extract can trigger the production of type I collagen, according to research in the *Journal of Ethnopharmacology,* possibly by triggering a protein that's important for the production of procollagen.[75]

Dong quai. Also known as female ginseng, this traditional Chinese herb has powerful benefits for skin. Studies show it decreases inflammation—and by now you know how devastating inflammation is for collagen—and reduces blood sugar, which also has anti-inflammatory benefits.

Astragalus. Astragalus root is a popular Chinese herb and has long been known to have skin-protecting benefits. Now research is beginning to reveal why: Astragalus stimulates hyaluronic acid production in the skin's fibroblasts, according to research in the *Journal of Ethnopharmacology,*[76] and hyaluronic acid in the skin binds with water to retain moisture and protect collagen.

The top six essential oils with blockbuster beauty benefits:

Frankincense. Research has shown that this ancient oil can reduce the appearance of scars and stretch marks, and it seems to have the same effect on wrinkles and fine lines, according to a paper in *Dermatologic Therapy*. In that study, researchers instructed study subjects to apply frankincense oil to one side of their face for thirty days. The treated side showed significant improvement in sun damage, skin texture, and fine lines as well as an increase in skin elasticity.[77] The secret behind its effectiveness is likely its inflammation-fighting ability. Mix two to three drops of the oil with equal parts coconut or jojoba oil and apply to your skin.

Pomegranate seed. The oil of the pomegranate seed offers powerful protection from sun damage, according to research, and actually inhibits the devastating UVB-induced damage, thereby protecting collagen.[78] Apply several drops to the skin before and after sun exposure.

Lavender. Research shows that lavender essential oil triggers the production of three of your body's most powerful antioxidants: glutathione (known as your body's master antioxidant), catalase, and superoxide dismutase. When cells are under stress, including fibroblasts, it's glutathione that comes to the rescue. Lavender oil is also helpful for wound healing, because it triggers protein synthesis, including collagen. Apply a few drops of lavender oil to the skin before bed; it also promotes sleep and reduces anxiety.

Myrrh oil. A powerful anti-inflammatory, myrrh oil contains terpenoids and sesquiterpenes, which control inflammation and also fight free radicals. Myrrh oil is part of my daily skin routine (and Chelsea's) because it also protects against the sun's damaging UV radiation and supports youthful, glowing skin. Apply a few drops to your skin before bed. (It will relax you, too!)

Jojoba. This isn't technically an essential oil, but I'm including it here because it is wonderfully hydrating, probably because it contains a number of helpful ingredients like vitamin E, vitamin B complex, silicon, chromium, copper, and zinc. It also can promote collagen, according to a study in the *Journal of Ethnopharmacology,* which showed that jojoba liquid wax, which is similar to oil, stimulated fibroblast synthesis of type I collagen in wounds.[79] Apply two to three drops of jojoba oil to your face.

Rosehip. There's a good reason this oil (which isn't actually an essential oil) has created a name for itself in the wrinkle-fighting realm: It's packed with vitamin C, which, as you already know, plays a vital role in collagen production. Not only that, it also is a rich source of essential fatty acids, including oleic, palmitic, linoleic, and gamma linoleic. It can strengthen nails, too. Apply a few drops to the areas you'd like to strengthen and support.

Protecting your skin isn't just a cosmetic issue. This vital tissue is the first layer of defense against invading pathogens as well as the largest organ in your body. Keeping it youthful and structurally sound has ramifications for your overall health—and promoting collagen is the single best strategy to safeguard your skin. But I don't want to trivialize the cosmetic impact of collagen. When you look in the mirror and see someone with vibrant hair and skin—which, by the way, can still be luminous (sometimes even more so!) if it has a few wrinkles and laugh lines—you feel better about yourself, which contributes to your happiness and sense of well-being. That, in turn, can help you be a better parent, partner, friend, and colleague. And there's nothing superficial about that.

CHAPTER 8

How Collagen and Other Remedies Can Heal Your Gut

The Most Effective Foods and Supplements for Transforming Digestive Health

Hippocrates, considered the father of modern medicine, said, "All disease begins in the gut." Indeed, before modern technology allowed us to identify the culprits underlying many illnesses, whether bacteria, a virus, or cancerous cells, doctors believed that a number of health issues were caused by imbalances in the gastrointestinal system. In that era, the word *hypochondria* (which literally means below, or "hypo," the rib cage, or "chondria") described not imagined illnesses but real physical ailments that could be traced to dysfunction in the GI tract.

With the advancement of technology, modern medicine veered away from the ancient view of the gut as an important source of disparate health problems.

Now, we're once again beginning to appreciate the fact that those doctors of old, whose practices were guided mostly by observation and instinct, were on to something. In fact, the science connecting your gastrointestinal health, particularly your small intestine, with the well-being of the rest of your body is growing exponentially by the day.

We now know, for instance, that the digestive tract is actually a vital immune barrier, protecting you from disease and contamination. The lining of the small intestine—colloquially known as your gut—has some especially tricky, and consequential, immunity-related responsibilities. It has to distinguish the foreign contents of the intestines from the body's own tissues, control the absorption of nutrients, and oversee the delicate balancing act between the local immune response and the trillions (yes, trillions!) of microbes that exist naturally in the gut. Altogether, a whopping 70 percent of your immune system response stems from the lining of your gut.

As long as it remains strong, the intestinal lining does a remarkable job. But when your body's physical defenses become overwhelmed by external factors—some of the biggies are stress, lack of sleep, toxins, viral or bacterial infections, or a low-fiber, high-sugar diet—the gut lining becomes vulnerable, making it easier for a population of unhealthy bacteria to gain ground and set up camp. And when that happens, it's honestly no exaggeration to say that all hell breaks loose.

When bad bacteria overwhelm the good they can create cracks and holes in the gut lining, disrupting the tightly controlled process of nutrient absorption and allowing partially digested food, toxins, and bugs to leak through. If those circumstances persist, you develop what's known as leaky gut syndrome, or increased intestinal permeability—a condition that we now believe affects millions of people in the United States. Worse, most sufferers don't even know they have it.

Leaky gut can cause food allergies, low energy, joint pain, thyroid disease, autoimmune conditions, and a sluggish metabolism. It interferes with nutrient absorption. It can lead to impaired digestion. And it has been linked to everything from Alzheimer's and anxiety to rheumatoid arthritis and type 2 diabetes. (My book *Eat Dirt* explains why leaky gut can cause a range of health problems—and how to cure it.)

At the same time, this dangerous intestinal permeability puts you at risk for common GI-related illnesses, like irritable bowel syndrome (IBS), inflammatory bowel disease (IBD), Crohn's disease, and chronic constipation, which affect up to 70 million people in the United States. It also plays a role in celiac disease, an autoimmune digestive disorder, in which the body mounts an immune reaction to gluten, a protein found naturally in wheat, barley, and rye. And these gastrocentric illnesses can wreak havoc on the rest of the body, triggering migraines, mood issues, fatigue, joint pain, and skin disorders, among other problems.

The health of your gut is another reason it's important to start consuming collagen. The connective tissue in your gut lining is made almost entirely of collagen, making it critical for digestive health. As a result, adding this long-overlooked substance to your diet helps tackle leaky gut at its source.

When you sip a cup of nourishing bone broth or add a scoop of hydrolyzed collagen to your green smoothie, your GI tract breaks down the substance into its constituent amino acids—including glycine, proline, and arginine (three of the key amino acids in collagen), which are essential for repairing and restoring the integrity of the intestinal lining. Indeed, collagen actually seals and heals this vital tissue, and as it does so it creates an environment in which a range of other health problems related to intestinal permeability can heal as well.

As I mentioned in the Introduction, I learned about the gut-healing benefits of collagen when I was a young doctor. I'd been recommending bone broth to patients, and it had been one of the cornerstones of the diet I created for my mom as she was going through her second bout of cancer. But I was busy and stressed, and I hadn't yet incorporated it fully into my own diet.

Then I started experiencing some health problems of my own. I usually have lots of energy, but I started feeling depleted and run-down, like I barely had the oomph to get through the day. I went to bed tired and woke up tired. It was awful. At the same time, I started having GI problems, with constipation one day and loose stool the next—completely out of character for me.

I saw an acupuncturist, because I knew that ancient healing treatment could help with fatigue and underlying imbalances in the body. He told me about powerful food combinations often used in traditional Chinese medicine to support digestive health, including "one-pot" recipes, like simmering healing herbs in meat and vegetable broths. From then on, I committed to incorporating those healing, collagen-rich dishes into my diet, and, as I did so, my gut symptoms began to clear up and my energy rebounded.

As I began doing my own research, I found dozens of case studies from Asia and the Middle East that provided persuasive evidence for how the consumption of collagen-rich broths, herbs, and spices could be deeply healing for the gut. I immediately started incorporating these time-tested health protocols into my treatment plans for patients, which gave me the opportunity to see innumerable examples of how people can benefit from these gut-healing tonics.

Research on the gut-related effects of collagen is still accumulating, but interest in the role this tissue plays in gastrointestinal illnesses, and, as a result, whole-body health, has never been higher. In the coming pages, you'll find a quick introduction to how and why your gut lining develops problems, a roundup of some of the intriguing research findings that reveal how collagen can help keep your GI system healthy and free of chronic symptoms, and a guide to the foods that can support collagen and gastrointestinal health. By taking steps to restore the stability of your gut lining, you'll see an improvement in numerous health conditions—and enable this important tissue to fulfill its destiny as the true health hero it is.

GETTING TO KNOW YOUR GUT LINING — AND WHY IT'S SO IMPORTANT

Most people don't give a second thought to the lining of their intestinal tract. But this unsung gatekeeper, buried deep inside your body, is a biological marvel. Inside its looping contours, food is broken down into its component parts and absorbed into the bloodstream, so the nutrients can be used by your body for fuel and routine maintenance.

This hardworking tissue, technically known as the mucosa, is made up of several layers:

- lamina propria, a layer of loose connective tissue that contains fibroblasts, which synthesize the collagen-rich extracellular matrix, as well as mesenchymal stem cells, plasma cells, and a variety of types of immune cells

- basement membrane (more on this tissue later)
- epithelium, or outer layer, the gatekeeper between the inside of your intestine and your bloodstream

All three layers of the gut mucosa interact and have important responsibilities for maintaining GI health. But the epithelium, which is made up of just one thin layer of cells, is the mainstay of the intestinal barrier. It is the tissue that determines whether your gut is leaky or not.

This single layer of epithelial cells is fixed firmly together by what are known as "tight junction" proteins—almost like numerous, infinitesimal suction cups that adhere each cell to its next-door neighbors. These tight junctions are the access points that allow substances to pass from your small intestine to your bloodstream. They allow healthful nutrients to pass through so they can heal and restore the rest of your body. But when the tight junctions become loose, as they do in people with leaky gut, they allow larger food molecules and microbes to sneak through and enter the bloodstream. Because the immune system identifies these larger molecules as foreign invaders, it forms antibodies to the particles, which not only can result in food allergies and sensitivities but also produces chronic inflammation—which, as I've mentioned before, is the root of dozens of modern-day diseases.

There are a number of ways your doctor can test for leaky gut, including blood and stool tests, but there are noteworthy signs that should make you consider whether leaky gut might be the cause of your health problems. Some of the symptoms, like bloating, fatigue, joint pain, headaches, and digestive problems, are so common they might not ring any alarm bells. But if you have several of those symptoms chronically, you should consider seeing a doctor who understands leaky gut. (Most functional medicine doctors are a good bet.) What's more, the condition can cause more glaring signals that are likely to get your attention. Here are the top seven problems that point strongly to an issue with your gut lining:

- *Food sensitivities.* Food allergies are one of the most common symptoms of leaky gut. As I mentioned above, when food particles and toxins seep through the intestinal barrier into the bloodstream, your immune system goes into overdrive and mass-produces a variety of antibodies, which may make you reactive to allergens, like gluten and dairy. In animal and human studies, leaky gut and food allergies have been linked. For instance, researchers at the Center for Celiac Research and Treatment at Massachusetts General Hospital have found that three factors are required for celiac to develop: ingestion of gluten, a genetic predisposition to celiac, and increased intestinal permeability.[80]

- *Inflammatory bowel disease.* As far back as 1988, scientists suggested that Crohn's disease might be more of a risk for people with leaky gut. Similarly, researchers have discovered that people with Crohn's disease and ulcerative colitis often have elevated gut permeability in their colons.

- *Autoimmune disease.* The key to understanding how leaky gut can cause an autoimmune disease is through the research on a protein known as zonulin, which opens up the tight junctions between the cells of the epithelial lining. Gliadin, a component of gluten, can increase zonulin levels, as can unhealthy gut bacteria. When the zonulin pathway runs amok, autoimmune and inflammatory disorders can occur in genetically susceptible people. Indeed, studies have shown that impaired intestinal epithelial function occurs before the onset of type 1 diabetes, an autoimmune disorder.[81] And animal studies have shown that inhibiting zonulin can ameliorate type 1 diabetes.[82] Likewise, when a certain type of bacteria slips through the tight junctions in those with leaky gut, it can cause lupus, an autoimmune disorder characterized by severe, persistent inflammation that leads to tissue damage in multiple organs.[83]

- *Thyroid problems.* There's evidence of a connection between leaky gut and Hashimoto's disease, an autoimmune thyroid disorder. Also known as chronic thyroiditis, this low-thyroid condition causes fatigue, weight gain, depression, and a host of other problems. As many as 40 percent of those with Hashimoto's have dilated tight junctions in their gut lining, according to a review in *Endocrine Connections*.[84] And when those gatekeepers become more lax, allowing an influx of unwanted pathogens to invade your bloodstream, your immune system goes into overdrive and starts attacking healthy tissues, including your thyroid.

■ *Nutrient malabsorption.* Because the small intestine is the place where nutrients are absorbed, when the gut lining starts failing and becomes inflamed, it functions less effectively. In my own patients with leaky gut, I observed a number of nutritional deficiencies, including vitamin B12, magnesium, and digestive enzymes. Malabsorption causes symptoms like weight loss, loss of muscle mass, weakness, difficulty concentrating and thinking clearly, and changes in your stool. Since those symptoms are often subtle, a stool test is the best way to diagnose the problem.

■ *Inflammatory skin conditions.* First described more than seventy years ago, the gut-skin connection theorizes that intestinal permeability can cause common skin conditions, including acne and psoriasis. Although the exact mechanism isn't clear, it's likely that the inflammation created by leaky gut negatively affects the skin as well.

■ *Mood issues and neurodevelopmental disorders.* You've probably heard of the gut-brain axis, the two-way communication that exists between the gut and the brain. But the gut and the brain don't just talk to each other. They influence each other; if one is unhealthy and functioning poorly, the other suffers as well. As a result, the toxins and inflammation caused by leaky gut can affect your mood and cognitive capacity. The inflammatory response characteristic of excess intestinal permeability triggers the release of pro-inflammatory cytokines and other chemicals that are thought to induce depression, for instance. And some experts theorize that autism may be connected to problems that arise in the gut microbiome, particularly within the first year of life.[85]

WHAT SCIENCE HAS REVEALED ABOUT COLLAGEN AND THE GUT

I've explained how and why the epithelial lining of the gut is important. But just below that thin layer of cells lies a dense sheet of specialized extracellular matrix known as the basement membrane — and I bet you can guess what it contains. Yep, *collagen*. In this case, it's type IV collagen, which is rich in the amino acids glycine, proline, and hydroxyproline as well as chains of a variety of other amino acids — an uncharacteristic pattern that allows this particular type of collagen to function as a membrane by assuming a lattice-like shape.

For years, scientists thought that basement membranes did little more than provide structural support.

Now we know that these membranes contain growth factors, which actually play a dynamic role in the tissues where they're found. They encourage cell development and rejuvenate nearby cells, and they're essential for the formation and effective functioning of the tight junctions between epithelial cells. In other words, they are vital for maintaining a healthy gut lining, as well as restoring its integrity when it becomes damaged. Likewise, the collagen-rich lamina propria provides support and nutrition for the epithelium, generates immune responses to protect the tissue, and helps with wound healing and tissue regeneration, thanks to its population of stem cells.

The latest research shows that gastrointestinal problems can be hard on collagen and its amino acids. When Canadian researchers analyzed the urine of people with IBS, the most commonly diagnosed gastrointestinal disorder in developed countries, they found metabolic evidence of collagen degradation—results they chalked up to the chronic low-grade inflammation caused by the illness.[86] Likewise, gastrointestinal levels of arginine, an amino acid in collagen, are decreased in people suffering from IBD.

However, collagen, and its amino acids, can also help fight GI problems. Getting more arginine, for instance, seems to help maintain normal intestinal physiology and facilitate healing of the gut lining when the intestine is damaged by IBD-related inflammation.[87] What's more, in mice with colitis, a form of IBD, arginine treatment helped reduce the permeability of the intestinal lining, thereby restoring its ability to do its job.[88] And when arginine was combined with glutamine, the two amino acids worked synergistically to slash pro-inflammatory cytokines in active Crohn's disease, another type of IBD.[89]

Research on a variety of gut-related illnesses is shedding light on the many ways in which collagen and the amino acids it contains can be beneficial for those with gastrointestinal issues. Here's a quick glimpse of some of those studies:

- *Collagen may bolster the tight junctions in the intestinal lining.* In a laboratory study, researchers from Tufts University induced dysfunction in samples of tissue from the intestinal lining and found that by administering marine collagen they were able to significantly mitigate the dysfunction by enhancing the integrity of the tight junctions.[90]

- *Glycine may alleviate damage to the intestinal lining—and seems to offer protection from IBD.* A study published in the *International Journal of Molecular Sciences* found that supplementing with glycine, the most abundant amino acid in the body, could heal some damage to the intestinal lining of piglets caused by *E. coli* infection.[91] At the same time, research that appeared in the journal *Gastroenterology* found that in animals with induced IBD, glycine administration alleviated diarrhea, weight loss, ulceration, and inflammatory changes in the colon, effectively pre-venting the illness from taking hold.[92] A review of gly-cine's effects by researchers at the University of North Carolina offered the most likely explanation for its gut-protecting effects: It's anti-inflammatory, it mod-ulates the local immune response, and it safeguards cells from harmful compounds.[93]

■ *Other amino acids in collagen can mitigate the dam-age caused by IBD.* A study in *Molecular Nutrition & Food Research* looked at rats suffering from IBD. When researchers gave the rodents a supplement of the amino acid hydroxyproline (one of the amino acids in the collagen in the intestinal basement membrane), it soothed the tissue damage caused by the illness.[94] There's evidence that glycine and prolyl-hydroxyproline may offer similar results in animals with colitis.

■ *L-glutamine stimulates the growth of the intestinal mucosa.* This amino acid is created by glutamic acid, an amino acid sometimes found in collagen. It is also in bone broth, and it works synergistically with the main amino acids in collagen. In fact, some research-ers believe that glutamine offers the strongest stimula-tion for epidermal growth of any nutrient. A study in *Journal of Parenteral and Enteral Nutrition* found that glutamine restores a protein that promotes tight junc-tions in patients with irritable bowel syndrome.[95] Other studies have found that glutamine deprivation can lead to leaky tight junctions.[96] And glutamine has been shown to preserve tight junction function during infection and other insults to the gut lining.[97]

■ *Collagen can protect your stomach, too.* A study published in *Research Communications in Molecular Pathology and Pharmacology* found that glycine can inhibit gastric secretion in the stomach and protect the mucus tissue from ulcers.[98]

■ *Finally, collagen helps with digestion.* As it moves through the GI tract, collagen attracts water and acid molecules. By the time it gets to the intestines it's filled with fluid, so it helps break down other proteins and carbohydrates and allows food to flow through the system more easily.

FOODS, HERBS, AND SUPPLEMENTS THAT SUPPORT COLLAGEN AND HEAL YOUR GUT

Reducing stress and exercising regularly are important for gut health. In fact, we now have forty years of research showing that stress negatively affects the microbial population in your gut. And research shows that stress makes the epithelial cells more permeable and erodes the thickness and quality of the mucus layer in general. Likewise, a variety of studies in animals and humans have shown that regular exercise can protect your gut. For instance, working out can encourage the growth of healthy microbes in your gut and increase the bacterial metabolite butyrate, which fosters epithelial cell proliferation and promotes gut barrier integrity.

But, unsurprisingly, diet plays an outsize role when it comes to the well-being of your GI system. While collagen alone will benefit your gut—especially when you consume it in the context of an anti-inflammatory diet—the following is a list of foods and supplements that have also been shown to be particularly helpful (and a few that are harmful) for your intestinal lining, as well as for the microbes in your gut.

Foods to eat:

- *Bone broth.* This therapeutic brew contains a hefty dose of the amino acids proline and glycine, as well as L-glutamine, all of which can help heal your damaged cell walls. As I mentioned above, dozens of studies have revealed that glutamine is a powerful weapon when it comes to protecting and improving gut health. It is not only beneficial in improving intestinal barrier structure and function but also can increase intestine-friendly bacteria, while decreasing dangerous microbes. (In addition to bone broth, glutamine is found in high quantities in grass-fed beef, spirulina, Chinese cabbage, cottage cheese, asparagus, broccoli rabe, wild-caught cod and salmon, venison, and turkey. You need at least three servings of glutamine-rich foods on a daily basis.)

■ *Fermented foods.* These superfoods rich in probiotics and organic acids help restore good gut flora, which improves nutrient absorption and overall gut health. Sauerkraut, kimchi, kvass, yogurt, and kefir are excellent sources.

■ *Coconut-based products.* The medium chain fatty acids in coconut are easier to digest than other fats, so they work well for those with leaky gut. Also, the fats found in coconut, including capric acid, caprylic acid, and lauric acid, have antimicrobial benefits. Coconut kefir is one of my favorite superfoods, because it provides both healthy fats and probiotics, which can help transform your digestive tract.

■ *Cooked vegetables.* This may surprise you, but people struggling with gut and digestive issues are better off consuming cooked, rather than raw, vegetables. The reason: Cooked vegetables, especially steamed, sautéed, and baked, are easier to digest—and they are still incredibly nutrient-dense and good for you. Traditional Chinese Medicine teaches that consuming asparagus, cauliflower, squash, pumpkin, and bitter veggies, like dandelion greens, radishes, and chard, can also promote digestive tract health by drying up dampness, along with candida (a type of yeast) overgrowth, which damages gut integrity.

■ *Healthy fats.* Egg yolks, avocados, coconut oil, ghee, and animal fats are easy on the gut and promote healing.

- *Omega-3 fats.* Anti-inflammatory foods like salmon, tuna, mackerel, halibut, black cod, sardines, and other wild-caught fish can benefit a damaged gut.
- *Fiber.* Research has shown that a low-fiber diet triggers the expansion of mucus-degrading bacteria in the gut. And as the thickness of the mucus begins to decrease, you become more susceptible to certain colitis-causing pathogens. That's why a diet rich in high-fiber foods, like sprouted chia seeds, flaxseeds, hempseeds, artichokes, broccoli, cauliflower, spinach, kale, blueberries, and raspberries, is crucial for gut health. If your gut isn't overly sensitive, aim for 30 to 40 grams of fiber a day.

Supplements that can support your gut:

- *Probiotics.* If you're going to take one supplement in addition to collagen to support your gut health, this is it. Probiotics help replenish good bacteria and crowd out the bad. Look for strains like *Bacillus clausii, Bacillus subtilis, Saccharomyces boulardii,* and *Bacillus coagulans.* Take 50 to 100 billion units a day.
- *L-glutamine.* Glutamine powder is anti-inflammatory and necessary for the growth and repair of your intestinal lining. I recommend buying l-alanyl-glutamine, because your body can absorb more of the substance when it comes in this form. For most people 2,000 to 5,000 milligrams a day is ideal.
- *Digestive enzymes.* These substances ensure that you're fully digesting your food, thereby decreasing

the likelihood that small food particles will escape through a leaky gut wall. Take one to two capsules at the beginning of each meal.

■ *Herbs and spices.* Consuming plant-based medicinal herbs can have a significant impact on your gut health. I recommend herbs that are anti-inflammatory and warming, a concept taken from Traditional Chinese Medicine. Herbs that bolster gut health and fall into that category include ginger, turmeric, and galangal. Also beneficial: herbs that dry up dampness and candida, including pau d'arco, parsley, jasmine, green tea, sage, and thyme. You can consume herbs with food, take them in capsule form, or steep them in hot water and drink as a delicious herbal tea.

■ *Licorice root.* This adaptogenic herb helps balance levels of the stress hormone cortisol and improves acid production in the stomach. At the same time, it supports the maintenance of the mucosal lining in the gut. Take approximately 500 milligrams once or twice a day.

■ *Lion's mane and reishi mushrooms.* These adaptogenic mushrooms have a positive effect on your gut—and your entire body. Lion's mane helps by healing the gut-brain connection. Studies have shown it reduces gut inflammation and stomach ulcers and helps regenerate nerve and brain tissue. Reishi has long been called the mushroom of immortality, and for good reason: It supports the immune system, the gut, and the adrenal glands, which secrete a variety of hormones that can impact the gut. Take the dosage prescribed on the supplement's label.

■ *Marshmallow root.* This natural antihistamine also has beneficial antioxidant activity. When it's used in conjunction with ginger, it helps protect your stomach from ulcers and offers overall support for gastrointestinal health. Take 500 milligrams once or twice a day.

■ *CBD oil.* This increasingly popular supplement contains cannabinoids found in the hemp plant, including cannabidiol (CBD), cannabinol (CBN), and cannabigerol (CBG), which have a calming effect on the sympathetic nervous system—and relaxing the nervous system can help heal the gut, soothe anxiety, and promote better-quality sleep (also good for GI health). For those with GI problems that are stress related, CBD oil is an effective supplement. Consume 20 to 40 milligrams daily.

Substances to avoid (or consume in moderation):

■ *Foods that feed the bad gut bacteria.* Added sugars, refined oils, genetically modified foods, synthetic food additives, and conventional dairy products all fall into this category. As a result, they can promote a runaway population of unhealthy microbes that overwhelm the protective bacteria—a condition that eventually leads to leaky gut.

- *Common gut toxins.* Everything from antibiotics to over-the-counter nonsteroidal anti-inflammatories to pesticides can affect the permeability of your gut. For instance, antibiotics kill off good bacteria and allow destructive microbes to gain ground. A study in the journal *Gut* found that patients developed increased intestinal permeability after taking NSAIDs for three to six months.[99] And pesticides in food can cause inflammation and wreak havoc with your hormones. Choose organic whenever you can.

- *Alcohol.* Both human and animal studies have come to the conclusion that long-term, heavy alcohol use can result in intestinal barrier dysfunction and alter the quality and quantity of gut bacteria. Although the exact mechanisms aren't entirely clear, studies have shown that the probiotic *Lactobacillus* is significantly suppressed during alcohol consumption. Likewise, alcohol converts to glucose in your body, and sugar is damaging to the epithelial lining. If you drink alcohol, it's best to buy certified organic or biodynamic, dry-farmed wines, which are free of mycotoxins, compounds produced by mold, and are lower in sugar and, as a result, produce less glucose in the body. A little alcohol won't hurt you. But try to steer clear of daily use, and avoid having more than one or two drinks on a single occasion.

It's easy to chalk up diarrhea, bloating, and gas to spoiled food or a passing bug. But there are good reasons to pay close attention to your bowel health and notice how different foods make you feel. The effects of mild celiac disease, for instance, can be subtle, but the consequences of missing an underlying gut problem can be devastating. Untreated, these gastrointestinal illnesses slowly erode your health, affecting everything from your mood to your energy level and your ability to function happily in the world.

My hope is that this chapter will serve as a wake-up call. By recognizing not only the importance of what's going on inside your belly but also how collagen can be pivotal for setting you on a path to better health, you're now officially ready to take control of your GI issues and improve your overall well-being.

CHAPTER 9

Collagen Secrets to Eliminate Pain and Inflammation

The Most Effective Strategy for Protecting Joints and Boosting Athletic Performance

Remember the information I shared in Chapter 6 about big-name professional athletes like Alex Rodriguez, Kobe Bryant, and Peyton Manning using stem cells to rejuvenate the collagen in the connective tissue around their joints? That is just one fascinating piece of a much larger — and rapidly expanding — story of the ways in which collagen can be *the* pivotal factor in keeping your joints healthy.

Joint health isn't just an issue for professional athletes. It affects everyone and matters for all of us — from the young, who want to preserve their springy, robust, and highly functioning tendons, cartilage, and ligaments, to recreational athletes and weekend warriors of every age, who want to continue participating in the activities they love for as long as they possibly can, to the growing population of mature and aged people, some of whom are living dangerously sedentary lives because they suffer from pain and disability due to loss of healthy connective tissue.

Between 2002 and 2014, the number of people who said they battled severe joint pain (rated seven or more on a scale of one to ten) jumped from 10.5 million to 14.6 million, according to the Centers for Disease Control[100]—and the numbers have almost certainly grown since then. About 54 million adults, by a conservative estimate, currently have medically diagnosed arthritis, the leading cause of joint pain, but by 2040, it's expected that some *78 million* adults in the United States—a quarter of the population!—will be struggling with the condition.[101]

Fortunately, collagen can provide much-needed relief no matter how severe the disease. And for those suffering with debilitating daily pain, it can be the secret ingredient that helps them regain their mobility, and along with it, their capacity to live independent, functional, engaged lives.

When Oregon resident Lora Stone, fifty-five, reached out to me not long ago, she told me that's exactly what happened to her. As a kid, she was a hard-core athlete and daredevil. "I raced dirt bikes and played three sports all through middle school and high school," she said. "When it came to fitness, I never learned to take it easy or be chill." Over the years she broke twenty bones, including several in her back. And then, as she got older, the pain set in. "I have arthritis in my hands, feet, knees, and back— and there are times when it has been debilitating," she said. "It got to the point where I couldn't really exercise anymore—and I don't do well with medications, so most of the time I just suffered."

That began to change in June 2017, when a friend recommended she try collagen supplements. "After three months of using a couple of scoops of multi-collagen protein every day, I had less pain in my back and joints, and they were no longer making the terrible grinding sounds I had grown used to," she said. "After a year of using collagen, my pain level was way down and my endurance and energy were higher than they'd been for a long time. My fingernails and my hair got healthier, too, and my gut problems have gone away. I still can't run, but I can move around without pain—and I can't tell you what a difference that has made in my life. Collagen has been a game-changer for me. I've recommended it to all my friends. I'll never stop taking it."

Lora's story echoes feedback I've heard from hundreds of patients, friends, and family over the years. Collagen's role in keeping your cartilage and connective tissue healthy is still underappreciated—although recognition of the substance's benefits is growing by the day. In the following pages, I'll explain more about the impressive body of scientific literature that is starting to reveal how, and why, collagen can bring relief to people like Lora—as well as how it can help anyone who has made fitness part of her or his life and wants to stay in the game for the long term.

MEET THE COLLAGENOUS TISSUE THAT PROTECTS AND CUSHIONS YOUR JOINTS

Most people know vaguely what connective tissue is, but they might be hard-pressed to define it. Here's a quick explanation: It's the stuff that binds, supports, or separates tissues and organs—and includes, as you'd expect, your cartilage, tendons, and ligaments, as well as some tissues that might surprise you, such as bones, fat, lymph, and blood. Bone is a dense type of connective tissue, for instance, while blood, lymph, and fat are more liquid, or viscous. But they come from the same embryological origin as other types of connectives—and they have similar functions in that they bind or connect disparate body parts.

Unlike your skin, which consists of cells that are tightly knit together with little "extracellular" space, connective tissue cells are dispersed in a gooey matrix. This viscous substance is made up of collagen, elastin, and fibroblasts (the cells that make collagen) as well as molecules known as glycosaminoglycans (GAGs) and proteoglycans, which are GAGs that are attached to proteins.

GAGs' primary role is to support and maintain collagen and elastin and help those fibrous substances retain moisture. GAGs are ideal molecules for lubricating the tissue around your joints, because they're gelatinous but not highly compressible. In other words, they allow for mobility and flexibility but offer a firm cushion that stands up to the many ways we bend, twist, and put pressure on our joints, like running, jumping, lifting, pushing, and pulling. GAGs contain glucosamine, a popular ingredient in joint supplements. There are a handful of specialized types of GAGs that are also helpful for joint health. You've probably heard of the following two types, which are found in your connective tissue and are crucial for its health:

- Hyaluronic acid (HA) is a type of GAG you've probably seen in popular skin care products. It's hot right now because it bolsters moisture retention, which, as you know, is fundamentally important to skin. But HA molecules are critical for joints, too. They're extremely large, as molecules go, which makes them excellent lubricators and shock absorbers in the connective tissue that buffers your joints.

- Chondroitin is another type of GAG found in cartilage and tendons. You've most likely seen it, in combination with glucosamine, in joint-supporting supplements. It's a vital component of connective tissue, because it enhances the shock-absorbing properties of collagen and blocks enzymes that break down cartilage.

Now that you understand a little about connective tissue in general, let's take a quick look at the types that are most relevant for joint health. Cartilage is the main connective tissue in your body. It's made up of closely packed collagen fibers in a rubbery, gelatinous substance called chondrin. It's strategically located throughout your body—in your nose, trachea, and ears, for instance—but the tissue that makes a difference for your mobility and ease of movement is in your joints.

A 2 to 3 millimeter layer of cartilage covers the bones that form each joint, whether in the shoulder, knee, hip, foot, ankle, elbow, hand, or wrist, serving as a pillowy shock absorber and lubricant that allows the bones to glide easily over one another as you move. Its unique combination of ingredients—a gel-like matrix filled with collagen that is up to 80 percent water (although that percentage decreases with age)— makes it a substance that creates very little friction, so it's the ideal material for protecting joints. The knee also contains a second type of cartilage, known as meniscus, that isn't actually connected to the bones but sits between them, providing extra stability and shock absorption.

The disks between your vertebrae are also made of cartilage. They're composed of a tough circular layer made of concentric sheets of collagen fibers and a gooey inner core, called the nucleus pulposus, that's a compression-resistant hydrated gel containing collagen, water, and proteoglycans. Positioned as they are between the bony vertebrae, the disks have three important jobs: They hold the spine together, allow for mobility, and absorb the impact that our daily activities place on our spinal column.

The tricky thing about cartilage is that it contains no blood vessels. Without a blood supply, it's difficult for the tissue to repair itself—and when cartilage wears away over time, whether due to injury, age, being overweight, or having poor postural alignment that places uneven pressure on the tissue, it can eventually lead to stiff, painful joints, the calling card of osteoarthritis.

However, by adding collagen to your diet, even tricky cartilage injuries can heal. My friend and colleague Jordan Rubin, a natural health practitioner and author of *The Maker's Diet,* learned how beneficial collagen can be when he developed crippling pain in his knee-cap in 2015. He was diagnosed with chondromalacia patella, or "runner's knee," which is caused by the breakdown of cartilage on the underside of the kneecap, or patella, allowing the knee and femur (the big bone in the front of your thigh) to rub together.

Here's what he told me about that time: "My knee became so tender and inflamed that I couldn't put weight on my foot without getting a jab of pain, and I couldn't straighten my leg. It was so bad I had to use crutches to get around. I already knew about bone broth, because I had used it successfully to heal Crohn's disease when I was in my twenties. By the time my knee pain came on, however, I had six children and had fallen out of the time-consuming habit of making it. But because bone broth contains copious amounts of collagen, a key component of cartilage, I recommitted myself to drinking six cups a day."

Within a few weeks, Jordan said, he had improved to the point where he no longer needed crutches. And here's what I love about bone broth as opposed to pharmaceuticals or anti-inflammatories: His knee continued to improve. Jordan calls it the crescendo effect. "With bone broth, health problems don't just heal. They become better than before," he said. "Now I'm forty-three, and part of my regular workout is doing squats with my son."

The two other main joint-related types of connective tissue, tendons and ligaments, are easy to confuse— and there are notable similarities. They're both made of collagen, and neither has an abundant blood supply, so healing can be slow. Both have a tendency to create dense scar tissue as they heal instead of youthful, supple tissue. But new research, which I'll explain below, is revealing how to avoid that.

Ligaments and tendons differ in important ways, too. Ligaments are x-shaped bands that attach bone to bone and help stabilize joints. They allow movement but also provide a limit, like a guardrail, so your joint mobility stays within a safe range. For instance, the anterior cruciate ligament (ACL) attaches the femur in your thigh to the tibia in your shin, keeping the knee stable while allowing for all the many movements the joint makes during the day. When pushed too far, of course, ligaments can tear; ACL tears, for instance, are common in athletes like basketball players and skiers.

Tendons, on the other hand, attach muscles to other body parts, usually bones. They have one of the highest tensile strengths of any soft tissue—an invaluable characteristic, considering the stress they're put under when we contract our muscles. But they're prone to injuries caused by overuse. The common, painful diagnosis of tendinitis is the result of inflammation or irritation of the tissue. While older adults are at risk for tendinitis because the elasticity of their tendons decreases with age, people of all ages can be plagued by the condition, from young dancers and computer gamers to office workers who type all day and avid tennis players. Other common tendon injuries are strains and tears.

When you think about all the activities we typically perform throughout the day—reaching for a tray on a high shelf, say, or running five miles or squatting repeatedly to pick up a toddler, or walking up and down stairs—you realize we expect a lot from our joints as well as the connective tissue that pads, lubricates, and protects them. It's not surprising that things can go wrong, especially as the tissues age and lose collagen and water, the keys to their strength and flexibility. But there's hopeful evidence that dietary collagen can help keep your connective tissue healthy—and heal it when things go awry.

THE SCIENCE THAT REVEALS HOW COLLAGEN PLAYS A ROLE IN JOINT HEALTH

In 1993, researchers from Harvard Medical School conducted a randomized, placebo-controlled trial of type II collagen in patients with rheumatoid arthritis, an autoimmune illness in which the body's own immune system attacks the lining of the joints, damaging cartilage and bone. Before the trial, all the participants were weaned off the immunosuppressive drugs they'd been taking. Then participants in the active arm of the trial were given type II collagen, the most abundant protein in cartilage, for three months, while the placebo group was given a sham supplement.

By the end of the trial, most patients in the collagen group had a significant decline in the number of swollen and tender joints as well as the severity of swelling and tenderness, while symptoms in the majority of those in the control group became more severe. In fact, the collagen users took fewer analgesics, on average, and their morning stiffness decreased, while their grip strength increased. Four of them had complete resolution of their disease.[102]

Even though this study, and others like it, began

showing that collagen could help with joint issues as far back as the 1990s, scientists were reluctant to give much credence to the approach, because they didn't believe that ingesting collagen would allow the amino acids to get to the places in your body that required help. Then, as I explained in an earlier chapter, researchers started slowly connecting the dots and building the case that consuming collagen does actually benefit the body.

First, Japanese researchers found the presence of high levels of a peptide containing hydroxyproline, a key amino acid in collagen, in the blood of people who had consumed a hydrolyzed collagen supplement. That 2005 study showed that collagen peptide levels increased in a dose-dependent manner, lending further credibility to the findings.[103]

Then, subsequent animal experiments showed that collagen peptide is deposited in skin after it leaves the blood.[104] At the same time, laboratory studies revealed that collagen peptides trigger the growth of fibroblasts (collagen-producing cells) in a collagen gel. And other research found that the peptides increase fibroblasts' production of hyaluronic acid and chondrocytes' production of glycosaminoglycan—revealing that they can affect joint tissue as well.[105]

Taken together, these findings strongly indicate that ingesting collagen can be beneficial for your joints. And thanks to that persuasive body of research, conventional wisdom about the effectiveness of the approach is in the process of undergoing a seismic shift, bringing more and more interest from researchers who are keen to find ways to safely treat common — sometimes debilitating — problems that affect far too many of us.

Here's a look at some of the promising findings:

- A randomized, double-blind, placebo-controlled study in *Complementary Therapies in Medicine* looked at two hundred people who were at least fifty years old and had joint pain in their lumbar spine or lower or upper limbs. More than half of those in the treatment group, who took 1,200 milligrams of hydrolyzed collagen a day for six months, experienced a significant alleviation of pain.[106]

- In a study of 250 patients diagnosed with osteoarthritis of the knee, Spanish researchers gave half of the group 10 grams of hydrolyzed collagen daily for six months. Compared to those who were given a placebo, participants in the collagen group had a significant decrease in pain as measured by two commonly used scales of joint pain — and those who had the greatest degree of joint deterioration actually benefitted the most.[107]

- U.K. researchers reported on the results of an interesting double-blind, randomized, placebo-controlled trial in 2018. They gave a supplement containing hydrolyzed fish collagen, glucosamine, chondroitin, L-carnitine, vitamins, and minerals to half of their 120 subjects, all of whom were between the ages of twenty-one and seventy; participants took the supplement for ninety days. While the researchers' primary objective was to see if there was a change in participants' skin elasticity (there was), the researchers also assessed joint pain in a subgroup of study subjects who were fifty-one to seventy years old. What they found: The collagen users' discomfort decreased, on average, 43 percent, while joint mobility increased by 39 percent. They concluded that the supplement could be "an effective solution to slow down the hallmarks of aging."[108]

- A 2018 review of studies on collagen for the treatment of osteoarthritis symptoms concluded that research convincingly shows that collagen is effective for decreasing joint stiffness as well as decreasing patients' self-reported pain levels.[109]

- And a paper in *PLOS One* may explain why the substance helps people suffering from osteoarthritis. In order to evaluate the tissue and cellular basis for the positive effects of collagen, researchers from the University of Rochester looked at mice that had developed osteoarthritis in response to a meniscus- and ligament-related injury. First, they supplemented the rodents' usual chow with collagen. Then, they took blood samples at various times and found elevated hydroxyproline levels — evidence that the collagen-related amino acid was circulating in their bloodstream. Finally, they harvested the rodents' joints to analyze the tissue, and here's what they discovered: The animals had dose-dependent increases in cartilage, chondrocyte number, and proteoglycan matrix at three and twelve weeks post-injury, leading the researchers to conclude that collagen is "disease modifying."[110] Not only does it protect cartilage and prevent cartilage cells from dying, but it also seems to have an anti-inflammatory effect on the injured tissue.

■ Meanwhile, a number of studies on rheumatoid arthritis (RA) have found positive results, including one published in *Arthritis Research and Therapy*. In that double-blind trial with 454 participants, researchers compared the effect of collagen with methotrexate, a commonly prescribed medication for RA, which is relatively safe at low doses but can be fatal if you take too much. They found that, while it wasn't quite as effective as methotrexate, collagen improved participants' pain, morning stiffness, joint tenderness, and swelling.[111] The bonus: Collagen is safe and free of side effects.

Researchers have also found increasingly promising results for the use of collagen in athletes with pain related to connective tissue and joints. In fact, the studies are so persuasive that the International Olympic Committee's 2018 consensus statement on dietary supplements gave a thumbs-up to the use of supplementation with gelatin or hydrolyzed collagen to increase collagen production, decrease pain, and help athletes recover from injuries.[112]

Here's a sampling of studies on athletes with connective tissue injuries:

- When German researchers conducted an observational study on the effect of 10 grams of hydrolyzed collagen on one hundred athletes with joint pain who did not have osteoarthritis, they found that 78 percent of participants reported a reduction of pain during movement by the end of the twelve-week study. Similar percentages of participants reported a decrease in pain when climbing stairs or carrying objects.[113]

- In a more rigorous follow-up of the above study, researchers at Penn State University conducted a randomized, placebo-controlled, double-blind study to assess the effects of collagen supplements in ninety-seven athletes who were having activity-related joint pain but had no evidence of joint disease. The results showed that participants who consumed 10 grams of collagen every day for twenty-four weeks improved on five parameters: joint pain at rest, when walking, when standing, when carrying objects, and when lifting.[114]

- Researchers at the Australian Institute of Sport published a paper in 2019 in *Nutrients* that looked at runners with Achilles tendinopathy, a difficult-to-treat condition that causes pain, swelling, and stiffness in the Achilles tendon, which connects your heel bone to your calf muscle. In their small, double-blind, placebo-controlled clinical trial, the researchers gave half of the participants a collagen supplement for three months and the other half a placebo; then, for another three months they swapped the protocol, so the placebo group got the collagen and vice versa. For the entire six months, both groups participated in a twice-daily calf-strengthening program, the traditional treatment for Achilles tendinopathy. The results showed that both groups improved significantly while they were consuming the collagen supplements—so much so that twelve of the eighteen participants were able to return to running—leading the researchers to conclude that the collagen supplement may accelerate the benefits of a calf-strengthening program.[115]

■ A paper published in the *American Journal of Clinical Nutrition* may help explain why collagen is helpful for athletic connective tissue injuries. In a small, randomized, double-blind trial, researchers divided subjects into three groups: One was given 5 grams of vitamin C–enriched gelatin (a form of collagen); the second was given 15 grams of the gelatin supplement; and the third was given a placebo. One hour after each group ingested the fluid, they jumped rope for six minutes. Participants repeated the pattern of supplementation and rope-skipping three times a day for three days, while researchers carefully monitored changes in their blood. At the end of the study, the data revealed that merely jumping rope for six minutes three times a day doubled the rate of collagen synthesis. And when participants consumed 15 grams of the collagen supplement, the rate of collagen synthesis doubled again. In other words, adding gelatin to a brief, intermittent exercise program improves collagen synthesis and, as the researchers put it, "could play a beneficial role in injury prevention and tissue repair."[116]

I mentioned in the last section that tendon and ligament injuries have a tendency to form scar tissue, as opposed to supple, new tissue, as they heal. But research indicates there's a way to circumvent that problem: By combining collagen with exercises targeted to the specific tissue you'd like to strengthen and/or heal. So, it makes sense to see a physical therapist to find the exercise protocol that's right for your condition. Short workout sessions seem to be the most effective for promoting connective tissue, according to research findings. Just take collagen or gelatin an hour before the workout, along with 200 milligrams of vitamin C, which stimulates collagen synthesis.

Given the results of studies in athletes and in those with joint-related disease, is it any wonder that more and more people are calling collagen the latest superfood?

THE FOODS THAT SUPPORT HEALTHY CONNECTIVE TISSUE

There are foods that can promote healing throughout the body, including connective tissue injuries and ailments. By making the right dietary choices, you can also keep cartilage, tendons, and ligaments strong and healthy—which will help you ward off common joint-related ailments.

Here are the joint-supporting all-stars.

The five foods (and categories of food) you can't live without:

Bone broth. I know I've talked about this a lot, but no chapter on connective tissue would be complete without a mention of this collagen-rich brew. Because here's the thing: Bone broth also contains a slew of other joint-healthy ingredients, like glucosamine and chondroitin as well as calcium, magnesium, phosophorus, silicon, and sulfur.

Sulfate-containing veggies. I mentioned these in Chapter 4, but to recap, foods like broccoli, cauliflower, garlic, cabbage, and onions contain sulfate, which combines with chondroitin to form cartilage. It's also required for the process of sulfation, to produce glucosamine sulfate and chondroitin sulfate, both of which help facilitate cartilage production and repair.

Bioflavonoids. Blueberries, blackberries, cherries, cinnamon, acai, red cabbage, and onions contain anthocyanidins, which help strengthen connective tissue by forming particular links between collagen fibers. And acai, apricots, nectarines, cherries, and raw cacao contain catechins, which prevent collagen degradation.

Zinc-containing foods. Lamb, grass-fed beef, oysters,

sesame seeds, and pumpkin seeds are all high in zinc, which is required for production of connective tissue.

Copper-containing foods. Avocado, cacao, sesame seeds, sunflower seeds, and cashews contain copper, which is required for the maturation of collagen.

The seven supplements you should consider adding to your diet:

Vitamin C. Not only does this substance increase collagen synthesis but it also accelerates bone healing after fractures and reduces oxidative stress. And it reduces the risk of cartilage loss and disease progression in people with osteoarthritis. When buying a vitamin C supplement, make sure to look for a food-based formula that contains superfoods like camu camu, amla berry, or acerola cherry. Take up to 1,000 millgrams of C per day.

Turmeric. I've already mentioned this potent anti-inflammatory a number of times, but it can protect connective tissue as well. Indeed, a number of studies in animals and in the lab have shown that it helps with rheumatoid arthritis, and here's why: Turmeric contains two joint-protecting compounds—curcumin, which reduces inflammation, and turmerone, which promotes stem cell growth. Together, they nourish and rejuvenate the tissue in your joints. Use turmeric liberally on food or take a supplement as directed.

Omega-3 fatty acids. The Arthritis Foundation recommends omega-3 fatty acids, and the fish, like salmon, tuna, sardines, and anchovies, that contain them, as part of an arthritis-fighting anti-inflammatory diet. And there's some evidence this all-purpose anti-inflammatory may be effective in helping fight pain. Consume 1,000 to 2,000 milligrams of an omega-3 supplement daily.

Hyaluronic acid. In high doses, this substance is so effective at treating osteoarthritis it has been approved by the Food and Drug Administration for that purpose. The FDA-approved version of HA requires injections from a health care provider — but there's evidence that lower doses, like those found in supplements, can reduce joint stiffness and chronic pain. Take a supplement as directed.

Glucosamine. Essential for the production of GAGs, glucosamine is also required for collagen and connective tissue formation and integrity. You can get this vital ingredient in bone broth or a bone broth protein supplement — or take a glucosamine-containing supplement as directed.

Chondroitin. A vital structural component of cartilage, chondroitin gives the tissue its bounce and compression resistance. Chondroitin is in bone broth and bone broth protein supplements, too — or you can take a chondroitin-containing supplement as directed.

Spirulina. This vitamin-rich supplement contains superoxide dismutase, an enzyme that helps reduce joint inflammation. Take a supplement as directed.

The four oils that fight pain and inflammation:

CBD oil. According to the Arthritis Foundation,

preliminary research suggests that CBD may help with arthritis pain.[117] In animal studies, for instance, CBD relieved arthritis pain and inflammation.[118] And a 2016 analysis of small studies in people with rheumatoid arthritis, osteoarthritis, and fibromyalgia (a chronic pain condition) found that CBD eased participants' pain and improved their ability to sleep.[119] CBD is a powerful anti-inflammatory and has no side effects, so it's worth a try. Take 20 milligrams of a certified organic CBD supplement two to three times a day.

Peppermint oil. This oil is often recommended for rheumatoid arthritis, because it has analgesic, anesthetic, and anti-inflammatory properties that help alleviate joint pain and stiffness. Rub a couple of drops onto the affected area.

Frankincense and myrrh oils. Each of these oils can be helpful for rheumatoid arthritis sufferers, but research has shown that when they're taken together, they can suppress joint inflammation and relieve pain in rheumatoid arthritis sufferers. Mix together and rub a couple of drops onto the affected area.

Joint health is an issue most of us don't consider till we have a problem, whether a sports injury or arthritis. And there's no doubt that once you've developed one of those issues, using collagen, along with collagen-bolstering nutrients, can help you fight it. But I'd like to propose another option before I wrap up this chapter: If we all proactively incorporated collagen into our diets, we could support the healthy levels of connective tissue we already have—and potentially prevent joint-related problems from ever occurring, or at least make them much less likely. Imagine that. What if we could avoid some of the million-plus hip and knee replacements in the United States every year? Or help keep older people active and engaged by keeping their joints pain-free? Or give midlife athletes the opportunity to return to play safely after a tendon or ligament injury?

By embracing collagen, I believe that this is not only possible but probable. I'll drink (a cup of bone broth) to that!

CHAPTER 10

Ten Other Surprising, Transformative Benefits of Collagen

Promoting Sleep, Detoxifying Your Body, Bolstering Immunity, and More

While collagen is becoming more widely known, especially in the realm of skin care and joint health, one of the reasons I wanted to write this book was to spread the word about its valuable effects that *aren't* talked about much yet—how collagen, and the amino acids in it, can help protect your cardiovascular system, for instance, and aid in weight loss, and even help you live a longer, healthier life. These intriguing benefits are hot areas of research in the scientific realm, but a number of the positive findings are only just starting to trickle out to the general public—and I'm excited to be able to share them with you here.

One of the reasons collagen can play such disparate roles in your body is because it's a protein—and proteins, and the amino acids they contain, are incredibly versatile. You might think that all they do is build muscle—or, in the case of collagen, provide structure and support to the surrounding tissue—but that's just part of their job.

Indeed, proteins have countless responsibilities in your body. They help produce hormones, the body's chemical messengers that allow cells in various parts of your body to communicate with one another; they facilitate important chemical reactions in your body; they help maintain your internal fluid and pH balance (the balance between acids and bases that is enormously important for your overall health); and they support your immune system by forming antibodies, the substances that protect you from all manner of viruses and bacteria and other disease-causing invaders.

And once you start looking at the amino acids in protein, things get even more interesting. Glycine, for instance, a predominant amino acid in collagen, is also a neurotransmitter, a chemical that transmits signals from one nerve cell to another, or to a muscle or gland cell. It can either stimulate or calm the brain and nervous system, so it is intimately involved in your body's everyday functioning and has been shown to be an effective sleep aid and memory enhancer.

As you begin your collagen journey, it makes sense for you to understand the *range* of ways this substance can make a difference in your health, including these compelling, but less well-known, outcomes. With that in mind, let's get right to it.

Research on collagen looks at the substance from a variety of angles. Some studies look at the effects of hydrolyzed collagen supplements given to people and animals. Others, like many of the studies on athletes with sports injuries that I mentioned in the previous chapter, use gelatin, a substance that is extremely similar to hydrolyzed collagen. And still others look at individual amino acids in collagen.

By now, you know that when you consume collagen, your body breaks it down into these amino acids. So studying these compounds can shed light on some of the nuanced benefits of collagen. And the latest research shows that collagen-related amino acids are powerhouse players in your physical and emotional well-being in their own right, with the ability to contribute to, and sometimes catalyze, meaningful health transformations.

Here are the top ten lesser-known—but truly mind-blowing—ways that collagen, and/or its amino acids, can be therapeutic.

COLLAGEN CAN IMPROVE SLEEP

One in four people in the United States develops insomnia every year, a condition characterized by an inability to fall asleep or stay asleep.[120] Chronic insomnia is defined as sleeplessness that strikes at least three nights a week and lasts for more than three months. Tossing and turning every few nights is so common it sounds innocuous. But it's not. Sleep deprivation raises your risk for depression, decreased work productivity, workplace accidents, and car accidents.

In addition, insomnia is difficult to treat. The medications that doctors often prescribe, like benzodiazepines and other sedatives, can be addictive if you take them night after night. They can make you feel groggy the next morning, and if you consume alcohol or other drugs at the same time, they can dangerously depress your nervous system—and sometimes cause you to stop breathing.

As a result, a side-effect-free approach for treating sleep problems is desperately needed—and research shows that glycine can help. For instance, a polysomnographic study, which tracked participants' brain waves, blood oxygen levels, heart rate, breathing, and eye movements throughout the night, found that glycine helped people fall asleep more quickly and enter deep sleep more quickly; indeed, participants' subjective reports the next day confirmed that they had slept better than usual, and their memories were sharper.[121] What's more, they felt less sleepy the next morning—results that echoed a similar small, randomized, placebo-controlled clinical trial published in *Sleep and Biological Rhythms*, which showed that participants who took 3 grams of glycine before bed at night were significantly more likely to say they felt more awake, lively, and clearheaded in the morning than those who took a placebo.[122]

My clinical experience supports those findings. I routinely recommended collagen to patients with gut problems or skin issues or joint pain. During our follow-up appointments, after they told me about the improvement they'd had with their primary problem, many of them would mention that they were sleeping better as well.

Animal studies point to a likely mechanism of action. When researchers gave rats oral glycine, they found that the substance showed up in the animals' cerebrospinal fluid and brain tissue, where it triggered the temperature-controlling part of the brain to drop the rats' core body temperature.[123] And that may be the key, or at least an important contributor, to glycine's effectiveness. Body temperature vacillates in a daily rhythm, rising in the morning and dropping at night. Research has long shown that as body temperature falls in the evening, it facilitates the onset of sleep as well as the ability to stay asleep. Since glycine seems to foster this drop, it can enhance restful slumber.

COLLAGEN CAN PROMOTE A CALMER, MORE UPBEAT MOOD

Anxiety disorders affect 40 million adults in the United States, or 18 percent of the population each year, and nearly half of the 16 million American adults diagnosed with depression have an anxiety disorder as well.[124] But sleep deprivation is a well-recognized contributor to depression and irritability—and difficulty falling asleep and staying asleep is a symptom of depression itself. Because glycine has the ability to help with sleep, it also has the potential to improve the emotional health and quality of life of millions of people.

This collagen-related amino acid also affects mood in ways that have nothing to do with sleep. In the brain stem and spinal cord, for instance, glycine acts as a soothing neurotransmitter, similar to GABA (gamma-aminobutyric acid), which plays a role in reducing anxiety and relaxing the nervous system. Indeed, a study in *Psychiatry and Clinical Neurosciences* found that oral glycine boosted serotonin, the brain chemical that is often low in people with depression, in the prefrontal cortex of rats.[125] The positive impact glycine has on serotonin may also benefit those with schizophrenia, although more research is needed to determine the substance's effectiveness.

Likewise, as I explained in detail in Chapter 8, collagen can give your gut the building blocks it needs to heal and seal itself. And the health of your gut is intimately linked to the health of your brain and to your mood. Ninety percent of your serotonin receptors are in your gut, for instance. At the same time, the teeming ecosystem of good and bad bacteria in your gut can also affect your mood. Recent research looking at two large groups of Belgians, for instance, found that several species of gut bacteria are missing in people with depression—and those species may play a role in the production of dopamine, a feel-good neurotransmitter in the brain, as well as butyrate, an anti-inflammatory, which could be connected, since inflammation has been implicated in depression.[126] The research, published in *Nature Microbiology,* doesn't prove cause and effect, but it expands on earlier animal research and smaller studies that have hinted at a similar gut-brain cause of depression.

COLLAGEN CAN HELP YOU CONTROL YOUR WEIGHT

We all know what a challenging national problem obesity is—and anyone who has tried to lose weight has learned that it's not easy. Hundreds of scientific studies have been devoted to finding the right combination of nutrients to make the process more successful—and high-protein diets consistently come out on top. Today, they're among the most popular diets in the United States, thanks to their reliable ability to help you shed pounds. Eating a protein-dense diet really does work.

One reason it's so effective is that protein is satisfying—and that applies to collagen just as it does to a nice pink salmon fillet. Food that keeps you full longer helps you eat less throughout the day. And there's evidence that hydrolyzed collagen protein is highly satisfying.[127] In fact, a number of participants in the Multi Collagen Makeover program mentioned how filling collagen is and said it had helped them control their appetites and slim down. I've experienced the same thing myself. My wife, Chelsea, and I rely on a daily dose of collagen in our morning smoothies to help us feel satisfied and energetic throughout the morning.

But that's just one of several interesting ways that collagen can help you shed pounds. For instance, a study on rats eating a high-sucrose diet (similar to the high-sugar diets many Americans consume) showed that glycine protected the animals from accumulating abdominal fat, which usually accrues when you eat a lot of sugar. Published in the *American Journal of Physiology—Regulatory, Integrative, and Comparative Physiology*, the research revealed that when they were given glycine, not only did the animals' fat cells shrink, but the rats also had a higher rate of fat metabolism[128]— a finding that has important implications extending beyond weight loss.

Deep abdominal fat is the toughest kind to shed *and* the most dangerous for your health, putting you at heightened risk of metabolic and cardiac problems. In fact, the rats on the high-sucrose diet without the addition of glycine developed high blood pressure and high triglycerides. So glycine may serve a dual purpose: By targeting the stubborn fat stored in your abdomen, it may help you lose weight *and* slash your risk of diseases that affect far too many overweight people around the world. As a result, it can be a game-changer for health.

When it comes to weight loss, one of the notable challenges many of us face is maintaining a slimmer body size. Studies confirm that most people experience this frustrating outcome: By diligently cutting calories, they lose weight fairly easily. But they struggle to keep the pounds off, even if they continue eating a low-calorie diet. One key reason this experience is so common is that when you shed pounds you typically lose lean muscle tissue along with fat. And, since muscle burns more calories than any other type of tissue in the body, your metabolic rate takes a nosedive.

Interestingly, collagen has a unique ability to help you maintain lean body mass as you drop pounds. In one study, researchers at the University of Melbourne looked at mice that were put on a calorie-restricted diet. When they gave the mice glycine, it not only accelerated their fat loss but also protected against muscle loss[129] — a finding that has been repeated in people with cancer and sepsis, two conditions in which sufferers often lose dangerous amounts of lean muscle as their weight plummets.

Glycine is known as the anti-aging amino acid because of its well-known ability to help your body maintain lean muscle mass into old age. The upshot: Adding collagen to your diet can protect your muscle tissue as you shed pounds—and help you keep the weight off for good.

COLLAGEN CAN BUILD STRONGER MUSCLE

Healthy muscle tissue can keep your metabolism humming along at a high rate—and contribute in myriad ways to your ability to stay happy and healthy with age. It can give you the physical stamina and agility to continue to travel, for instance, or go to community or cultural events, or participate in physical activities with your children or grandchildren; it can allow you to bounce back more easily after illnesses and injuries; and it can help you maintain a high energy level so you can continue to meet the demands of your job, even as the years tick by.

Robust muscle and connective tissue is particularly important for athletes, and the International Olympic Committee's 2018 consensus statement on dietary supplements and high-performance athletes lists collagen and gelatin in its section on supplements that may assist with training capacity, recovery, muscle soreness, and injury management.[130]

Collagen seems to be particularly helpful when paired with exercise. In a study in the *British Journal of Nutrition,* fifty-three elderly men with muscle loss underwent three supervised resistance-training sessions a week for twelve weeks. Roughly half were given a collagen supplement, and the other half received a placebo. At the end of the trial, all participants' muscle mass, bone mass, and quadriceps strength increased, while their fat mass decreased—but the effect was significantly more pronounced in those who received the collagen supplements.[131]

These findings make a lot of sense, when you consider that muscle is suffused with collagen, where it provides mechanical strength and immune support and helps repair the tissue. In fact, research indicates that hydroxyproline-glycine plays a role in muscle cell differentiation and growth. And, as you learned in the previous section, glycine has been found to help inhibit the deterioration of muscle protein.

But here's something I didn't mention: Glycine can also aid in muscle building. Turns out, this tiny amino acid is required to synthesize creatine, a compound that helps repair damaged muscle and build new, stronger tissue. Athletes often use creatine supplements to boost strength, endurance, and overall performance. In fact, one seminal study found that when you add creatine supplements to your usual strength-training regimen, you can double your strength and lean muscle gains.[132] So getting glycine in your diet can bolster your ability to create this valuable muscle-building substance naturally.

And there's another collagen-related amino acid that's important for healthy muscle tissue. Arginine has the ability to significantly increase growth hormone levels, which contributes to muscle growth. It also is known to effectively improve blood flow, so your body can deliver more nutrients and oxygen to muscle tissue. And feeding your muscle allows you not only to build more healthy tissue but also to exercise more efficiently with less fatigue and pain.

That can be great for all of us—but it can be truly life-changing for people who have narrowing of the blood vessels in their legs and feet, a condition that makes it painful to walk. As a result, sufferers are at risk of becoming dangerously sedentary. Here's the good news: Research shows that arginine supplementation can improve walking distance and reduce muscle aches in patients with this type of atherosclerosis[133]—so it can help them maintain muscle and stay healthy and active in spite of their disease.

COLLAGEN CAN PROMOTE BONE HEALTH

About 50 percent of bone is made up of protein, and the majority of it is collagen. Indeed, people who consume too little protein have reduced bone density and increased rates of bone loss. That's more important than it may sound at first blush. It's estimated that one in three women and one in five men over age fifty will fracture a bone due to osteoporosis—and those fractures can be devastating. Australian and Danish researchers recently reported on a ten-year study in people over fifty who had sustained fractures related to fragile bones. In the first year after breaking a hip, 33 percent of men and 20 percent of women had a higher risk of dying—and the risk was still significant a full decade later.[134]

Happily, protein can be particularly beneficial for aging people, who are at the most risk of osteoporosis. A study of more than 140,000 postmenopausal women, for instance, found that each 20 percent increase in protein intake was associated with significantly higher bone mineral density throughout their bodies, including in the fracture-prone hips.[135]

What's more, animal studies looking specifically at collagen protein have shown that it can increase bone formation and bone mineral density (BMD)—and a study published in *Nutrients* in 2018 found the same thing happens in postmenopausal women with age-related low bone density. In that randomized, placebo-controlled trial, women taking collagen supplements for a year had significantly increased bone density in their spines as well as their femoral necks, the bone at the top of the femur that is most likely to break when someone fractures their hip, whereas BMD decreased over the same time period in the placebo group. Collagen supplementation was also associated with a favorable shift in biological markers that are indicative of increased bone formation and reduced bone erosion.[136]

Similarly, a study in pairs of identical twins, who have the same genetic makeup and, as a result, are often used in scientific research, revealed that in each pair of twins, the one with the higher intake of glycine and alanine, another collagen-related amino acid, had significantly higher BMD in her or his spine than the sibling with lower intake;[137] that finding is particularly hopeful for people with a family history of osteoporosis, because the research indicates that upping your consumption of glycine and alanine may improve your bone health, regardless of your genetic risk for the condition.

COLLAGEN CAN BE HEALTHY FOR YOUR HEART

Cardiovascular disease is listed as the underlying cause in about one out of every three deaths in the United States. An average of one person in the country dies every thirty-eight seconds of the disease, according to recent stats from the American Heart Association.[138] So finding ways to support heart health and the cardiovascular system as a whole is high on the national agenda. Now, more and more researchers are looking to collagen as a potential way to achieve this goal.

Not long ago, Norwegian researchers reported on a study in which they followed more than four thousand people who had experienced angina, or chest pain, for nearly seven and a half years. The results, reported in the *Journal of the American Heart Association,* showed that those with higher glycine levels in the blood had a lower prevalence of obesity, high blood pressure, and diabetes—all contributors to cardiovascular disease. As important, those with higher glycine had a decreased risk of having a heart attack during the study period. The researchers theorized that glycine's positive effects on heart health could stem from the fact that the amino acid might help the body metabolize and get rid of fats and cholesterol.[139]

But there are other ways glycine likely bolsters cardio-vascular health. Research has shown, for instance, that in rats eating a high-sucrose diet, increasing their intake of this amino acid decreases their levels of circulating fatty acids, abdominal fat, and blood pressure.[140] At the same time, glycine deficiency can be dangerous. There's evidence that it fosters atherosclerosis in mice[141]—and low glycine levels correlate with obesity and diabetes. On the flip side, when insulin resistance improves, so do plasma glycine concentrations.[142]

Arginine, too, has earned kudos for its positive effects on heart health. Indeed, one of the most noteworthy benefits of arginine is its ability to improve blood flow and circulation. In the body, this amino acid is converted into nitric oxide, which causes blood vessels to dilate, thereby keeping your blood pressure within a normal range. And high blood pressure is a major risk factor for stroke. Indeed, a literature review published in the *Journal of Chiropractic Medicine* confirmed that arginine helped reduce diastolic and systolic blood pressure in people with hypertension.[143]

There's also evidence that it prevents clots and plaque from forming—another way it reduces the risk of stroke. And, like glycine, arginine can be helpful for those with angina, because nitric oxide prevents clots that cut off blood supply. Taken together, it's safe to say that having healthy glycine and arginine levels—which you can sustain by adding collagen to your diet—can protect your heart.

COLLAGEN CAN STRENGTHEN YOUR IMMUNE SYSTEM

A healthy immune system is obviously vital to your ability to fight off colds and other viruses as well as battle cancer and random cellular abnormalities. And, as you know by now, the majority of your immune system resides in your gut—which means that keeping your belly healthy can keep your whole body healthy. What's more, fascinating research has begun to show that the amino acids in collagen may help keep this disease-fighting system in tip-top shape. Indeed, not long ago, a woman named Raquel sent me this note:

"Four years ago, I had a new baby and was feeling ill. I caught every sickness that came along. I went to almost fifteen doctors and no one could tell me what my problem was. Then, I came across your website and read about leaky gut. I tried collagen, and now I know how to treat my problem. I have no words to thank you."

Scientific research supports the collagen-immunity link. A study in rats with deteriorated immunity caused by the drug methotrexate found that giving them type II collagen for twenty-eight days bolstered their body weight as well as key markers of immunity, including T cells, which were significantly increased in the blood and spleen.[144]

T cells are a type of white blood cell that plays a primary role in fighting cancer, as well as bacterial and viral invaders. (They're called T cells because they mature and develop in your thymus, located behind your sternum.) In a laboratory study reported in the journal *Cell,* researchers found that by elevating levels of arginine, an amino acid in collagen, they could bolster T cells' metabolic fitness and survival capacity — and in mice arginine enhanced the cells' anti-tumor activity.[145] At the same time, researchers have long suspected that glycine has the ability to modulate the immune system and may also play a yet-to-be-explained role in fighting cancer.

Arginine can bolster immune function as well, thanks to its free radical–scavenging ability. And, since nitric oxide acts as a neurotransmitter and protective agent against outside threats, it has a positive effect on both the central nervous system and the immune system.

COLLAGEN CAN INCREASE ANTIOXIDANT PROTECTION AND DETOXIFICATION

Glycine is one of three amino acids that your body requires to produce glutathione—and, as I've mentioned in previous chapters, glutathione is a superhero antioxidant, offering cells protection from damaging free radicals. But glutathione does more than that. It also helps support immune function and may help prevent the progression of cancer; improves insulin sensitivity, which helps prevent the development of type 2 diabetes; generates sperm cells; reduces symptoms of Parkinson's disease; and protects the body from the damage caused by ulcerative colitis. Some researchers speculate that it may even help children with autism, since there's evidence that they have lower levels of the substance than children without autism.

At the same time, glutathione can detoxify chemicals that make their way into your body, like environmental toxins and pollutants and prescription and recreational drugs. In fact, doctors intentionally bolster the substance in people who overdose on acetaminophen. The reason: In the liver, glutathione binds to toxins, the first step in escorting them out of the body. Research in people who frequently eat fish shows that those who have genes that tamp down glutathione synthesis have higher levels of mercury.[146]

Unfortunately, levels of glutathione drop with age, so as the years tick by, it's more important than ever to have high levels of the substance's building blocks, including arginine, cysteine, and glutamate. A study published in the *American Journal of Clinical Nutrition* found that although glutathione deficiency in elderly people occurs because of a notable reduction in synthesis, supplementation with glycine and cysteine fully restores the body's glutathione production system.[147]

COLLAGEN CAN RESTORE SEXUAL AND HORMONE HEALTH

As men age, their ability to develop and maintain an erection begins to deteriorate. Roughly 40 percent of men are affected by this concerning condition by age forty, and 70 percent develop a problem by the time they're seventy.[148] Doctors have long known that nitric oxide, which, as you already know, is bolstered by arginine, is necessary for healthy erections. Men with cardiovascular problems tied to low levels of nitric oxide in the blood are more likely to suffer from erectile dysfunction (ED). The reason: An erection depends on the ability of the smooth muscle to relax, a process triggered by nitric oxide.

Given the fact that arginine supports nitric oxide, researchers have been exploring whether the amino acid can help men who are struggling with ED. A study in the *Journal of Sex & Marital Therapy* found that, while arginine alone was only mildly effective at combating ED, when it was combined with pycnogenol, another name for the extract of French maritime pine bark, it helped 92.5 percent of men achieve a normal erection after three months of treatment.[149] In fact, arginine seems to improve circulation to the genital tissues in both men and women, making it an effective way to turn around sexual performance problems for both sexes.

Additionally, some research suggests that treatment with N-acetyl cysteine and arginine together can help balance hormones and restore normal sexual function in women with estrogen imbalance as well as polycystic ovary syndrome, a common health problem caused by an imbalance of reproductive hormones, and a leading cause of infertility. A small pilot study indicated that when women who are struggling to conceive consume arginine, along with herbs like chasteberry, green tea extract, and antioxidant supplements, rates of pregnancy improve.[150]

COLLAGEN MAY INCREASE YOUR LIFE SPAN — AND YOUR HEALTH SPAN

In the realm of anti-aging science, the most sought-after outcome is the ability to extend longevity. One of the most effective and hopeful strategies for achieving that goal is through fasting and/or calorie restriction. But recent cutting-edge research on amino acids has revealed an additional strategy that might be helpful: supplementing with glycine.

A study in *PLOS Genetics,* for instance, looked at *C. elegans,* a tiny nematode that is often used in scientific research. Although it's a simple organism, many of the molecular signals that control its development are also found in humans, and studying cell death in the worm could hold the key to understanding—and counteracting—the effects of aging in humans. In fact, in this study supplementing with glycine significantly prolonged the life span of *C. elegans.*

Similar research found that glycine supplementation extends the lives of mice and rats as well. Anti-aging researchers from around the country collaborated on one of the recent papers showing that glycine could extend the lives of mice and concluded, "Our glycine results strengthen the idea that modulation of dietary amino acid levels can increase healthy life span in mice, and provide a foundation for further investigation of dietary effects on aging and late-life diseases."[151]

Meanwhile, glycine's positive effects on glutathione

may help you remain healthy well into old age. In a study published in the *Journals of Gerontology: Biological Sciences*, researchers followed nearly 2,600 people age sixty and older living in Stockholm. For six years, they logged participants' chronic conditions and tracked their total serum levels of glutathione.[152] What they found: As glutathione levels dropped, the number of diseases the study subjects fell prey to increased, findings that point to the idea that propping up glutathione levels by taking glycine, one of the components of glutathione, can keep you healthy even as you get up in years.

Indeed, the title of a separate study published in the *American Journal of Clinical Nutrition* may sum it up best of all: "Deficient Synthesis of Glutathione Underlies Oxidative Stress in Aging and Can Be Corrected by Dietary Cysteine and Glycine Supplementation."[153] Collagen may be one of your best allies in your quest to age well.

Individually, each of these discrete effects of collagen is important. Taken together, the vast array of evidence is jaw-dropping. For a substance we've ignored for the past hundred or so years, collagen is quickly proving itself to be worthy of admission into the esteemed pantheon of superfoods. I'm glad you've decided to welcome it into your life and hope that by reading this far you have a thorough understanding of the many reasons I recommend it and use it daily.

The next few chapters will give you all the practical information you need for incorporating collagen into your diet. Before we leave this informational section of the book, I want to thank you again for taking this journey—and congratulate you on the one you're about to begin. Here's to reaping the dramatic and diverse benefits of collagen in your own life!

PART III

The Collagen Diet Plan

CHAPTER 11

The 3-Day Collagen Cleanse

Everything You Need to Know to Do an At-Home Collagen-Based Reset

You've probably heard a lot about cleanses in the last few years, and you may have even come across some that require you to shell out a shocking amount of money for juices or other special ingredients. The collagen cleanse isn't like that. It's a simple, no-gimmicks approach that allows you to take advantage of two incredibly powerful health-transforming strategies: intermittent fasting and collagen loading.

Intermittent fasting is a strategy in which you eat during a prescribed window during the day—usually six, eight, or ten hours—so your body has a longer-than-usual stretch without food. (You might have your first meal at noon and your last at 8 p.m., for instance.) Even that fleeting fast can, according to a study in *Obesity*, activate molecular signaling pathways that "optimize physiological function, enhance performance, and slow aging and disease processes."[154]

Fasts and cleanses are slightly different, but the collagen cleanse actually uses both strategies. A fast is when you abstain from a type of food, or from all food, for a certain period of time. A cleanse is a dietary strategy that supports detoxification. Collagen is great for cleansing, because it contains glycine, which plays a role in the production of glutathione, and, as I explained in Chapter 10, glutathione binds to toxins in the liver and helps your body excrete them. Additionally, the herbs, fruits, and veggies you'll be consuming on the collagen cleanse support and enhance this necessary cleaning-out process.

Indeed, in just three days, the collagen cleanse can help you lose weight, normalize blood sugar, decrease cholesterol, promote growth hormone (which helps you burn fat and create more collagen-rich body tissues), help you think more clearly, slash inflammation, reset hunger hormones to healthy levels, slow the aging process, and possibly even add years to your life. Its benefits stem from both its super-healthy ingredients and the fasting aspect. In fact, research has shown that intermittent fasting, like long-term fasting, prompts your cells to make more copies of the SIRT3 gene, one of several longevity genes and one that prevents free radical formation and improves cells' ability to repair damage they incur through contact with toxins and daily wear and tear.[155]

Intermittent fasting has been shown to be so effective at promoting beneficial hormonal and metabolic changes in your body that the National Institutes of Health has funded a number of studies to determine how and why it works—and dozens of books have recently been written about the approach. That makes it sound trendy, but in truth fasting has been practiced by cultures around the world for thousands of years. It's a fundamental part of many religious traditions and has long been recognized as a way to cure and rejuvenate the body. Philippus Paracelsus, a Swiss physician who lived in the 1500s, said, "Fasting is the greatest remedy; the physician within." Even Benjamin Franklin was a fan. He said, "The best of all medicines is resting and fasting."

My wife, Chelsea, and I do a collagen cleanse that includes intermittent fasting at least twice a year—and I've recommended it to hundreds of patients—because it's a quick and efficient way to clean out your system and restore lost nutrients. I always feel refreshed and rejuvenated afterward.

Because you'll be sticking with liquids only while you fast, you'll reduce the usual amount of stress on your digestive system; just as sleeping at night gives your body time to undertake fundamental repairs, reducing your food intake gives your GI system the opportunity to rest and repair. And the nutrition you *will* be putting into your body is manifestly healing.

A cornerstone of the approach is bone broth, one of

the most nutrient-dense, therapeutic foods known to man. As a result, you'll be loading up on collagen. So this fast is not only an effective way to launch your new collagen-friendly lifestyle, but it also confers tons of collagen-driven benefits in its own right.

As you've already learned, bone broth and other collagen-rich foods and supplements can reduce symptoms of common digestive disorders, like leaky gut syndrome, irritable bowel, or inflammatory bowel disease; it can support healthy joints, ligaments, and tendons; it can strengthen your bones; it can boost your immunity by increasing the beneficial bacteria in your gut; and it can halt and even turn around the obvious signs of skin aging.

Some cleanses fail to provide the important trace minerals we need for ongoing energy, immunity, digestion, and cellular repair, and because they're often lacking in electrolytes they can cause brain fog, fatigue, and moodiness. But because bone broth is made from animal bones, tendons, skin, and cartilage — tissues that are teeming with minerals and electrolytes, like calcium, phosphorus, magnesium, sodium, potassium, sulfate, and fluoride — the risk of those problems is far lower. Indeed, the glycine in bone broth (and other forms of collagen) can help you get more sleep, which is a salve for mood, and may also enhance mental performance and memory.

Another benefit of doing a collagen-based fast: While you can lose weight, just as you can anytime you drastically reduce your caloric intake, adding collagen can prevent the muscle loss that often accompanies fasting-related weight loss. Because collagen is made up of the amino acids glycine, proline, arginine, hydroxyproline, and glutamic acid, which shore up muscle, this 3-day cleanse can help you hang on to every ounce of your healthy, calorie-burning tissue, even as you drop pounds. At the same time, glycine is a necessary ingredient for the production of glutathione, one of the body's most powerful detoxifying agents, which helps the liver flush out chemicals, stored hormones, and other waste.

Juice is another aspect of this collagen cleanse that's particularly important. Simply put, juicing is an easy way to get a whopping helping of fresh veggies, herbs, spices, and low-sugar fruit into your diet in one easy meal. In liquid form, veggies and herbs are super easy to digest, allowing your body to quickly absorb more of the vitamins and minerals they contain. Drinking raw, freshly made juice can increase your intake of antioxidants and nutrients, such as chlorophyll, a green pigment found in certain plant foods that is beneficial for detoxification and controlling inflammation. At the same time, raw juice is packed with antioxidants that fight free radicals, setting the stage for maximum absorption and utilization of the dietary collagen you're consuming, and protecting your body's current stores of collagen.

The best and easiest way to make homemade raw juices is with a juicer; however, if you don't own a juicer, you can place the ingredients in a high-speed blender, blend so that everything is as liquefied as possible, then strain out the solid pulp. To save time, make at least two servings of juice at once and store the leftovers in the fridge; they'll keep for up to two days, but you'll probably drink it before then. If you're truly pressed for time, instead of juicing you can mix water with a powdered green superfood supplement. Do not substitute with store-bought juice, however; it's loaded with sugar and, sometimes, preservatives.

In the coming pages, I provide some delicious, nutrient-packed juice recipes, but if you want to get creative, feel free! Here are some of the detoxifying, collagen-boosting veggies, herbs, and fruit I use regularly, any of which you can use in your own concoctions:

- beets
- blackberries
- cabbage
- carrots
- celery
- cilantro
- cucumber
- ginger
- kale
- lemon
- lime
- mint

- parsley
- raspberries
- romaine lettuce
- spinach
- Swiss chard
- turmeric
- wheatgrass

The third pillar of my collagen cleanse is herbal tea. Tea has been used as a health supplement and medicinal substance in both Traditional Chinese Medicine and Ayurvedic medicine for four thousand years. For instance, a homemade tea that contains cinnamon, pau d'arco (a medicinal substance that comes from the wood and bark of the pau d'arco tree), ginger, and astragalus can turn around candida overgrowth. A brew made from milk thistle, turmeric, bupleurum, and moringa can help with detoxification. A combination of schisandra, holy basil, matcha, and white tea can help with aging skin. Simmering ginger, peppermint, licorice, and astragalus together can bolster gut health. And a tea made of ginger, echinacea, astragalus, clove, and reishi mushrooms can support your immune system. For the purposes of this cleanse, you can try making some herbal teas on your own; just boil two cups of water, then add a teaspoon of your favorite herb or spice, be it tulsi (holy basil) or turmeric powder. Or keep it super simple and use organic, packaged herbal teas of your choice. If you like a little caffeine, green tea is a great option; excellent decaf choices are ginger or chamomile.

In addition to giving your digestive system a break, the reason we do cleanses with fluids—and these fluids in particular—is that broth, veggie juice, and herbal tea are "serum soluble." That means your bloodstream and cells can easily absorb them, so the nutrients they contain make their way quickly and efficiently into your body, where they can be utilized in whatever way you most need them.

Anyone can benefit from a collagen cleanse, but you can expect to reap particularly noticeable benefits if you suffer from digestive disorders or symptoms like bloating, diarrhea, or constipation; food allergies; or fatigue, sluggishness, or difficulty sleeping.

During your collagen cleanse, stick to the following guidelines every day:

- Consume only liquids, including bone broth, raw juice made mostly from veggies (but you can include a single type of fruit), teas, herbal infusions, coffee, and water. These liquids will provide essential nutrients and decrease hunger—and the bone broth, juice, and herbal tea will keep you hydrated.
- Get two servings of collagen, with one serving from real bone broth (homemade or store-bought—so long as it's *real* bone broth—or made from a hydrolyzed bone broth supplement and water). The other

serving can be from a hydrolyzed collagen supplement, preferably one that contains multiple types of collagen.

- Drink at least two cups of herbal tea or herbal infusions.

- Have two cups of antioxidant-providing raw juice that's made mostly of veggies.

- Drink two to four cups of water.

- If you're so inclined, have a cup or two of black coffee—but no more than that, and steer clear of it after noon; otherwise it may interfere with your sleep.

- Listen to your body! While intermittent fasting has loads of benefits, if you feel weak, light-headed, or fatigued, have an extra raw juice with a serving of collagen protein; if that doesn't help, have a light snack, like a cup of steamed veggies, an avocado, or a handful of blueberries.

As I mentioned above, intermittent fasts usually restrict calorie consumption to a six-, eight-, or ten-hour window, so choose the one that's right for you. If you're new to fasting and cleanses, I suggest you start with the eight-hour time frame; if that's too difficult, you can stretch it to ten hours and add another veggie juice or collagen dose at 8 p.m. Or, if you have experience, you can be more restrictive in your eating hours, while still consuming two servings of collagen, veggie juice, and herbal tea. But give yourself the flexibility to change it up if you feel it's too difficult. Also, pick the hours that work best with your lifestyle. Some people like to eat from 10 a.m. or 12 p.m. to 6 p.m. Others prefer to shift their window earlier or later. You can have water or black coffee outside of your eating window and remain in a fasted state; your window doesn't start until you consume something with calories.

If you exercise, you'll get the biggest fat burn if you do so in a fasted state, so lots of people choose to work out in the morning before they've eaten. Regardless of when you exercise, plan to have a cup of bone broth or a green juice with some hydrolyzed collagen protein immediately afterward, so you can replenish your calories and prevent a precipitous drop in energy.

Ready to begin? Here's a complete guide to your 3-day collagen cleanse, using an eight-hour eating window.

Day 1

Upon waking
- Water and, if desired, black coffee, matcha, or herbal tea

10 a.m.
- Veggie juice: cucumber, beets, Swiss chard, lemon, and turmeric

12 p.m.
- Cherry Vanilla Collagen Smoothie (see the recipe on page 250)
- Herbal tea or infusion (2 tea bags)

3 p.m.

- Veggie juice: celery, cucumber, spinach, cilantro, lime, and ginger

6 p.m.

- Homemade bone broth (or broth made from a bone broth protein supplement)
- Herbal tea or infusion

Day 2

Upon waking

- Water and, if desired, black coffee, matcha, or herbal tea

10 a.m.

- Veggie juice: spinach, romaine lettuce, beets, cucumber, lemon, and turmeric

12 p.m.

- Strawberry Coconut Bone Broth Smoothie (see the recipe on page 254)
- Herbal tea or infusion

3 p.m.

- Veggie juice: raspberries, cabbage, carrots, ginger, wheatgrass, mint, and lemon

6 p.m.

- Homemade bone broth (or broth made from a bone broth protein supplement)
- Herbal tea or infusion

Day 3

Upon waking
- Water and, if desired, black coffee, matcha, or herbal tea

10 a.m.
- One scoop hydrolyzed collagen protein mixed with a glass of water, almond milk, or unsweetened coconut milk

12 p.m.
- Veggie juice: cucumber, spinach, blackberries, lemon, ginger, and parsley

3 p.m.
- Homemade bone broth (or broth made from bone broth protein supplement)

6 p.m.
- Veggie juice: carrot, cabbage, kale, Swiss chard, lime, and cilantro
- Herbal tea or infusion

CHAPTER 12

The 28-Day Collagen Diet Meal Plan

Your Step-by-Step Guide to Bringing Collagen into Your Life

Welcome to the heart of your collagen journey! I'm delighted you're here. What lies ahead is a way of eating that can shield you from the most common challenges of aging, from wrinkles and thinning hair to arthritis, gastrointestinal ailments, cardiovascular problems, and weakened immunity. What's more, it's simple—and sustainable.

Now that you've completed your 3-day cleanse, your body is well on its way to becoming a collagen-building machine—and you're ready to embark on the super-nutritious diet you'll find in the coming pages. Although this can be a short-term diet, it's also one you can easily tweak—and stay on for years. Built around the healthiest inflammation-fighting ingredients, it's carefully designed to support whole body wellness—*and* keep your collagen levels high. It also provides amino acid balance, something you've likely been missing your whole life. And it can help you lose weight.

Every day, you'll be consuming the equivalent of three (or more!) servings of collagen from a variety of sources. Bone broth and hydrolyzed collagen supplements are the mainstays of this approach. But I also encourage you to bolster your collagen consumption by eating the skin on chicken and fish and adding organ meats to your diet.

If you have time, I recommend making bone broth at home. Here's how: Put several pounds of beef bones or chicken necks, feet, and wings, along with carrots, celery, onion, garlic, and your favorite herbs and spices, in a stockpot with 18 to 20 cups of water; simmer for 24 to 48 hours. If you don't have the time or bandwidth to make your own, fear not; easier alternatives are available. You can make bone broth from a powdered supplement, as I've mentioned, or buy it premade from your health food store. Regardless, you'll find it to be an incredibly versatile health food. As you'll see from the fantastic recipes in Chapter 13, you can add grains, legumes, veggies, or protein to bone broth—or use it as a base for stews or smoothies. As you get more comfortable with the program, feel free to get creative with it—and have fun. Food is meant to be savored and enjoyed.

By eating several servings of collagen a day, you'll

not only be receiving a healthy balance of amino acids but also consuming nearly 25 to 30 grams of protein, which will fill you up and offer sustained energy. But many of you will benefit from having more than three servings of collagen. If you're over forty, or already have problems with your joints, GI system, metabolism, or skin, or you exercise more than an hour a day, I suggest you consume four or five servings, which will ensure that you're ingesting enough amino acids to repair and rebuild your collagen-rich tissue.

You can eat collagen throughout the day, but there are several times that are ideal—and may help you get the most from your efforts. Here's when I like to have collagen:

- First thing in the morning. Adding collagen to your coffee or breakfast smoothie will give you a solid hit of protein to start your day; as a result, it will fill you up and fuel your body for the next few hours.

- After exercise. As with any other protein supplement, it's helpful to consume collagen after a workout, because it promotes tissue repair and muscle growth. In addition, the unique amino acids in collagen are the building blocks of the soft tissue in your joints, which may have experienced stress during your workout—so a post-workout dose of collagen gives your cartilage, tendons, and ligaments the nutritional support they need to undergo necessary maintenance as well.

- Before bed. As you've already learned, collagen is teeming with glycine, the amino acid that has been shown in scientific studies to help you fall asleep and stay asleep. Research shows that 3 to 5 grams of glycine is enough to encourage peaceful slumber. Since glycine makes up about a third of collagen, one heaping scoop of a hydrolyzed collagen supplement, or a half cup of bone broth, will provide what you need.

By adding collagen throughout the day you'll likely be taking in more protein than usual, so this eating plan is great for curbing hunger and cravings—and losing weight. The bonus: Diets with higher amounts of protein also support healthy blood sugar levels.

Some of you undoubtedly already eat relatively nutritious diets; for you, adopting my collagen plan may feel more like tweaking your current approach than making wholesale changes. For others who are used to consuming more processed foods, this way of eating, which includes an abundance of vegetables, healthy fats and oils, protein, and unprocessed carbohydrates, will feel more foreign. As a result, it may be more challenging to stick with it.

If you run into emotional resistance and find yourself craving processed foods, here's what I want you to think about: Recently, researchers from the National Institutes of Health looked at people eating an ultra-processed diet (with foods like sugary cereal and packaged blueberry muffins with margarine for breakfast, or canned chicken salad sandwiches on white bread with canned peaches in heavy syrup for dinner) versus those eating an unprocessed diet (with meals like plain Greek yogurt with strawberries, bananas, and walnuts for breakfast and stir fry with beef, broccoli, onions, peppers, ginger, garlic, and olive oil over basmati rice for dinner). The study subjects stayed at the NIH Clinical Center's Metabolic Clinical Research Unit for twenty-eight days, so the researchers knew exactly what they ate, and how much, at every meal. One half of the group was given the ultra-processed diet for the first two weeks, then switched to the unprocessed diet for the next two weeks, while the other half did the reverse. Participants were given three meals a day, plus snacks, and were instructed to eat as much or as little as they liked. The meals in the two groups varied widely by how processed they were, but the foods that were included were matched for energy density and basic macronutrients.

Here's what the research revealed: The group eating the processed diet consumed a whopping *500 calories* a day more than the unprocessed diet group, on average. Unsurprisingly, the processed diet group gained an average of about two pounds in two weeks, while the unprocessed group lost about two pounds.[156]

It's one of the most persuasive diet studies I've ever seen, because it effectively links processed foods with weight gain, which, in turn, contributes to everything from arthritis and GI problems to heart disease and high blood pressure. I wanted to share it with you here, because it's a graphic illustration of the risks of processed foods—and the rewards of consuming a diet that's based around whole foods from nature.

While the NIH study diet didn't contain collagen, it was in other respects very similar to the diet I provide in these pages. And, as you've learned by now, a varied diet that includes an abundance of healthy plant and animal foods will provide your body with the essential nutrients it requires, including vitamin A, vitamin C, copper, sulfur, and iron, to properly absorb—and make use of—dietary collagen.

And don't forget to focus on adopting healthy lifestyle strategies as you eat your way to a healthier you. The following strategies can enhance the benefits of this life-changing diet plan:

- Maintain your usual water intake, ideally around eight 8-ounce glasses a day. Maintaining fluid intake is important, because it aids in digestion—and thirst often masquerades as hunger. If you're hungry, have a glass of water and wait ten minutes to see if the feeling subsides.

- Aim to get at least seven hours of sleep every night. Sleep gives the healthy nutrients you're ingesting during the day time to repair your organs, muscles, and collagen-rich tissues. Sleep boosts your mood and energy as well—and will help you stick to this diet plan.

■ Exercise as you normally would—and if you don't exercise, please start. If you're typically sedentary, start doing twenty minutes of walking every day. If you're used to exercising, save your tough workouts for days when you're not fasting. On fasting days, it's best to stick with walking or yoga.

■ Don't beat yourself up if you stray from the plan a little. One of the most common reasons people give up on a diet is that they cheat. They mistake a single slipup or two for wholesale failure. Don't let that happen to you! Try to avoid consuming empty calories from processed or prepackaged foods. But if you have a moment of weakness, don't let it derail your whole plan. Just acknowledge the mistake—and use it as a moment to recommit to the program.

With that in mind, let's get to it.

THE 28-DAY COLLAGEN DIET MEAL PLAN

Day 1

Breakfast
- *Cherry Vanilla Collagen Smoothie* (page 250)
- Organic coffee (optional: blended with 1–2 tablespoons of coconut oil, butter, or ghee) or tea/herbal infusion of your choice

Lunch
- *Butternut Bisque* (page 258)
- Side salad topped with homemade dressing: 1 tablespoon of olive oil mixed with apple cider vinegar and seasoned to taste
- *Golden Tea* (page 249)

Snack (optional)
- *Guacamole* (page 297) served with raw veggies

Dinner
- 6 ounces of wild-caught salmon (or another type of wild-caught fish) cooked in 1 tablespoon of coconut or olive oil
- Steamed broccoli or brussels sprouts, topped with 1 tablespoon of flax oil and seasoned to taste
- ½ baked sweet potato
- Tea/herbal infusion of your choice

Day 2

Breakfast
- *Peach Probiotic Smoothie* (page 253)
- Organic coffee (optional: blended with 1–2 tablespoons of coconut oil, butter, or ghee) or tea/herbal infusion of your choice

Lunch
- *Indian Curry Soup* (page 263)

- Side salad topped with homemade dressing: 1 tablespoon of olive oil mixed with apple cider vinegar and seasoned to taste
- Tea/herbal infusion of your choice

Snack (optional)
- 4 ounces of strawberries served with ½ cup full-fat cottage cheese

Dinner
- *Spaghetti Squash with Roasted Chicken, Lemon, and Parsley* (page 272)
- ½ cup of fermented veggies (such as sauerkraut or kimchi)
- Side salad topped with homemade dressing: 1 tablespoon of olive oil mixed with apple cider vinegar and seasoned to taste
- Tea/herbal infusion of your choice

Dessert
- *Key Lime Pie* (page 306)

Day 3

Breakfast
- *Strawberry Coconut Bone Broth Smoothie* (page 254)
- Organic coffee (optional: blended with 1–2 tablespoons of coconut oil, butter, or ghee) or tea/herbal infusion of your choice

Lunch

- *Beef and Butternut Squash Soup* (page 257)
- ½ cup of fermented veggies
- Tea/herbal infusion of your choice

Snack (optional)

- *Blueberry Muffins* (page 294)

Dinner

- *Roasted Chicken with Roma Tomatoes and Onions* (page 271)
- *Maple-Glazed Rosemary Carrots* (page 288)
- Tea/herbal infusion of your choice

Day 4 (Optional Cleanse Day)

Breakfast

- *Carrot Ginger Bone Broth Shake* (page 252)
- Organic coffee (optional: blended with 1–2 tablespoons of coconut oil, butter, or ghee) or tea/herbal infusion of your choice

Lunch

- *Green Brain-Boosting Smoothie* (page 250)
- Organic coffee (optional: blended with 1–2 tablespoons of coconut oil, butter, or ghee) or tea/herbal infusion of your choice

Snack

- Tea/herbal infusion of your choice

Dinner

- Whole Body Tonic Juice: 4 celery stalks, ½ cucumber, 1 cup pineapple chunks, ½ green apple, 1 cup baby spinach leaves, 1 lemon, and 1-inch knob ginger
- Bone broth soup (or 1 scoop of bone broth protein mixed with 1¼ cups hot water)
- Tea/herbal infusion of your choice

Day 5

Breakfast

- *Blueberry Bliss Collagen Smoothie* (page 251)
- Organic coffee (optional: blended with 1–2 tablespoons of coconut oil, butter, or ghee) or tea/herbal infusion of your choice

Lunch

- *Slow Cooker Gingered Beef and Broccoli Soup* (page 262)
- Side salad topped with homemade dressing: 1 tablespoon of olive oil mixed with apple cider vinegar and seasoned to taste
- Tea/herbal infusion of your choice

Snack (optional)

- *No-Bake Bone Broth Protein Muffins* (page 298)

Dinner

- Leftover *Roasted Chicken with Roma Tomatoes and Onions* (page 271)
- Leftover *Maple-Glazed Rosemary Carrots* (page 288)
- Tea/herbal infusion of your choice

Dessert

- *No-Bake Cashew Truffles* (page 307)

Day 6

Breakfast

- *Collagen-Enhancing Veggie-Loaded Egg Bake* (page 255)
- Organic coffee (optional: blended with 1–2 tablespoons of coconut oil, butter, or ghee) or tea/herbal infusion of your choice

Lunch

- *Leafy Green Salad with Salmon* (page 277)
- *Sweet Potato Fries* (page 291)
- Tea/herbal infusion of your choice

Snack (optional)

- 4 ounces of blueberries served with ½ cup full-fat cottage cheese

Dinner

- *Slow Cooker Steak Fajitas* (page 284)
- Tea/herbal infusion of your choice

Day 7

Breakfast

- *Pumpkin Pie Smoothie* (page 253)
- Organic coffee (optional: blended with 1–2 tablespoons of coconut oil, butter, or ghee) or tea/herbal infusion of your choice

Lunch

- Leftover *Slow Cooker Steak Fajitas* (page 284)
- Tea/herbal infusion of your choice

Snack (optional)

- *Butternut Squash Chips* (page 295)

Dinner

- 6 ounces of organic free-range chicken cooked in 1 tablespoon of olive or coconut oil
- Summer squash or zucchini sautéed in 1–2 teaspoons of olive oil, coconut oil, or ghee
- Tea/herbal infusion of your choice

Day 8

Breakfast

- *Loaded Kefir Breakfast Bowl* (page 256)
- *Collagen Coffee* (page 249)

Lunch

- *Creamy Tomato Soup* (page 261)
- ½ cup of fermented veggies

- Side salad topped with homemade dressing:
  1 tablespoon of olive oil mixed with apple
  cider vinegar and seasoned to taste
- Tea/herbal infusion of your choice

Snack (optional)
- 4 ounces of raspberries served with ½ cup
  full-fat cottage cheese

Dinner
- *Quinoa-Stuffed Bell Peppers* (page 275)
- *Mashed Faux-tatoes* (page 289)
- Tea/herbal infusion of your choice

Day 9

Breakfast
- *Mint Chocolate Smoothie* (page 252)
- Organic coffee (optional: blended with 1–2
  tablespoons of coconut oil, butter, or ghee)
  or tea/herbal infusion of your choice

Lunch
- 6 ounces of organic grass-fed lamb cooked in
  1 tablespoon of coconut oil
- Steamed kale topped with 1 tablespoon of
  olive oil and seasoned to taste
- ½ cup of quinoa or rice cooked in bone
  broth (optional: sprinkle with turmeric and
  herbs)
- Tea/herbal infusion of your choice

Snack (optional)
- *Blueberry Macadamia Bars* (page 293)

Dinner
- *Stir-Fry Salmon* (page 279)
- *Mashed Sweet Potatoes* (page 290)
- Tea/herbal infusion of your choice

Dessert
- *Apple Crisp* (page 301)

Day 10

Breakfast
- *Black and Blue Berry Smoothie* (page 251)
- Organic coffee (optional: blended with 1–2 tablespoons of coconut oil, butter, or ghee) or tea/herbal infusion of your choice

Lunch
- Leftover *Stir-Fry Salmon* (page 279)
- ½ cup of fermented veggies
- ½ avocado
- Tea/herbal infusion of your choice

Snack (optional)
- Leftover *Blueberry Macadamia Bars* (page 293)

Dinner
- *Meatball Soup* (page 264)

- ½ cup of quinoa or rice cooked in bone broth (optional: sprinkle with turmeric and herbs)
- Side salad topped with homemade dressing: 1 tablespoon of olive oil mixed with apple cider vinegar and seasoned to taste
- Tea/herbal infusion of your choice

Day 11 (Optional Cleanse Day)

Breakfast
- *Cherry Vanilla Collagen Smoothie* (page 250)
- Organic coffee (optional: blended with 1–2 tablespoons of coconut oil, butter, or ghee) or tea/herbal infusion of your choice

Lunch
- *Peach Probiotic Smoothie* (page 253)
- Tea/herbal infusion of your choice

Snack
- Spicy Heart Health Juice: ⅛ or less jalapeño, 1-inch knob ginger, 1 clove garlic, 1 medium raw beet, 2 carrots, 1 lemon, and 1 cucumber

Dinner
- Immune-Supporting Juice: 1 bell pepper (red, green, yellow, or orange), 1 small head broccoli (with stem), 1 lemon, 1 cucumber,

1-inch knob ginger, and 1 tablespoon apple cider vinegar
- *Green Brain-Boosting Smoothie* (page 250)
- Tea/herbal infusion of your choice

Day 12

Breakfast
- 2–3 eggs fried in 1 tablespoon of butter or avocado oil
- Organic coffee (optional: blended with 1–2 tablespoons of coconut oil, butter, or ghee) or tea/herbal infusion of your choice

Lunch
- *"Noodle" Bowls* (page 265)
- *Cauliflower Tabbouleh Salad* (page 286)
- Tea/herbal infusion of your choice

Snack (optional)
- Raw veggies served with ½ cup hummus

Dinner
- *Chicken Noodle Soup* (page 260)
- *Roasted Cruciferous Vegetables* (page 290)
- Tea/herbal infusion of your choice

Dessert
- *Banana Chia Pudding* (page 302)

Day 13

Breakfast
- *Strawberry Coconut Bone Broth Smoothie* (page 254)
- Organic coffee (optional: blended with 1–2 tablespoons of coconut oil, butter, or ghee) or tea/herbal infusion of your choice

Lunch
- Leftover *Chicken Noodle Soup* (page 260)
- Leftover *Cauliflower Tabbouleh Salad* (page 286) or ½ baked sweet potato
- Tea/herbal infusion of your choice

Snack (optional)
- 4 ounces of blueberries served with ½ cup full-fat cottage cheese

Dinner
- 2–3 eggs fried in 1 tablespoon of butter or avocado oil
- Sliced tomato and cucumber drizzled with lemon juice and olive oil and seasoned to taste
- Tea/herbal infusion of your choice

Day 14

Breakfast

- *Pumpkin Pie Smoothie* (page 253)
- Organic coffee (optional: blended with 1–2 tablespoons of coconut oil, butter, or ghee) or tea/herbal infusion of your choice

Lunch

- 4 ounces of organic grass-fed beef cooked in 1 tablespoon of coconut oil
- Steamed or roasted asparagus drizzled with 1 tablespoon of olive oil and seasoned to taste
- ½ cup of brown rice cooked in bone broth and topped with turmeric and herbs of your choice

Snack (optional)

- *Almond Cacao Collagen Balls* (page 292)

Dinner

- 6 ounces of organic free-range chicken cooked in 1 tablespoon of coconut oil
- *Mashed Faux-tatoes* (page 289)
- ½ cup of fermented veggies

Day 15

Breakfast

- *Black and Blue Berry Smoothie* (page 251)
- Organic coffee (optional: blended with 1–2 tablespoons of coconut oil, butter, or ghee) or tea/herbal infusion of your choice

Lunch

- *Butternut, Cauliflower, and Carrot Soup* (page 259)
- Side salad topped with homemade dressing: 1 tablespoon of olive oil mixed with apple cider vinegar and seasoned to taste
- *Golden Tea* (page 249)

Snack (optional)

- Leftover *Almond Cacao Collagen Balls* (page 292)

Dinner

- 6 ounces of wild-caught salmon (or another type of wild-caught fish) cooked in 1 tablespoon of coconut or olive oil
- Steamed broccoli or brussels sprouts topped with 1 tablespoon of flax oil and seasoned to taste
- ½ baked sweet potato
- Tea/herbal infusion of your choice

Day 16

Breakfast
- *Collagen-Enhancing Veggie-Loaded Egg Bake* (page 255)
- Organic coffee (optional: blended with 1–2 tablespoons of coconut oil, butter, or ghee) or tea/herbal infusion of your choice

Lunch
- Leftover *Butternut, Cauliflower, and Carrot Soup* (page 259)
- Side salad topped with homemade dressing: 1 tablespoon of olive oil mixed with apple cider vinegar and seasoned to taste
- Tea/herbal infusion of your choice

Snack (optional)
- 4 ounces of strawberries served with ½ cup full-fat cottage cheese

Dinner
- *Chicken Tenders* (page 269)
- ½ cup of fermented veggies
- Side salad topped with homemade dressing: 1 tablespoon of olive oil mixed with apple cider vinegar and seasoned to taste
- Tea/herbal infusion of your choice

Dessert
- *Coconut Chia Pudding* (page 305)

Day 17

Breakfast
- 2–3 eggs fried in 1 tablespoon of butter or avocado oil
- Organic coffee (optional: blended with 1–2 tablespoons of coconut oil, butter, or ghee) or tea/herbal infusion of your choice

Lunch
- Leftover *Chicken Tenders* (page 269)
- ½ cup of fermented veggies
- Tea/herbal infusion of your choice

Snack (optional)
- *Chocolate Cherry Protein Bars* (page 296)

Dinner
- *Shepherd's Pie* (page 281)
- Side salad topped with homemade dressing: 1 tablespoon of olive oil mixed with apple cider vinegar and seasoned to taste
- Tea/herbal infusion of your choice

Day 18 (Optional Cleanse Day)

Breakfast
- *Blueberry Bliss Collagen Smoothie* (page 251)

- Organic coffee (optional: blended with 1–2 tablespoons of coconut oil, butter, or ghee) or tea/herbal infusion of your choice

Lunch
- *Mint Chocolate Smoothie* (page 252
- Organic coffee or tea/herbal infusion of your choice (optional)

Snack
- Tea/herbal infusion of your choice

Dinner
- Whole Body Tonic Juice: 4 celery stalks, ½ cucumber, 1 cup pineapple chunks, ½ green apple, 1 cup baby spinach leaves, 1 lemon, and 1-inch knob ginger
- Bone broth soup (or 1 scoop of bone broth protein mixed with 1¼ cups hot water)
- Tea/herbal infusion of your choice

Day 19

Breakfast
- Omelet made with bell peppers, spinach, and tomatoes
- Organic coffee (optional: blended with
- 1–2 tablespoons of coconut oil, butter, or ghee) or tea/herbal infusion of your choice

Lunch
- Leftover *Shepherd's Pie* (page 281)
- Side salad topped with homemade dressing: 1 tablespoon of olive oil mixed with apple cider vinegar and seasoned to taste
- Tea/herbal infusion of your choice

Snack (optional)
- Leftover *Chocolate Cherry Protein Bars* (page 296)

Dinner
- *Quinoa-Stuffed Bell Peppers* (page 275)
- ½ cup fermented veggies
- Tea/herbal infusion of your choice

Dessert
- *No-Bake Chocolate Chip Cookies* (page 307)

Day 20

Breakfast
- *Strawberry Coconut Bone Broth Smoothie* (page 254)
- Organic coffee (optional: blended with 1–2 tablespoons of coconut oil, butter, or ghee) or tea/herbal infusion of your choice

Lunch
- *Butternut Bisque* (page 258)

- Side salad topped with homemade dressing:
  1 tablespoon of olive oil mixed with apple
  cider vinegar and seasoned to taste
- Tea/herbal infusion of your choice

Snack (optional)
- 4 ounces of blueberries served with ½ cup
  full-fat cottage cheese

Dinner
- *Seared Tuna with Asparagus* (page 280)
- *Bean Salad* (page 285)
- Tea/herbal infusion of your choice

Day 21

Breakfast
- *Loaded Kefir Breakfast Bowl* (page 256)
- Organic coffee (optional: blended with 1–2
  tablespoons of coconut oil, butter, or ghee)
  or tea/herbal infusion of your choice

Lunch
- Leftover *Seared Tuna with Asparagus* (page
  280)
- *Sweet Potato Fries* (page 291)
- Tea/herbal infusion of your choice

Snack (optional)
- *Guacamole* (page 297) served with raw
  veggies

Dinner

- 6 ounces of organic free-range chicken cooked in
  1 tablespoon of olive or coconut oil
- Summer squash or zucchini sautéed in
  1–2 teaspoons of olive oil, coconut oil, or ghee
- Tea/herbal infusion of your choice

Day 22

Breakfast

- *Peach Probiotic Smoothie* (page 253)

Lunch

- *Beef and Butternut Squash Soup* (page 257)
- ½ cup of fermented veggies
- Side salad topped with homemade dressing:
  1 tablespoon of olive oil mixed with apple cider vinegar and seasoned to taste
- Tea/herbal infusion of your choice

Snack (optional)

- 4 ounces of raspberries served with ½ cup full-fat cottage cheese

Dinner

- *Italian Chicken and Eggplant Casserole* (page 268)
- *Roasted Cruciferous Vegetables* (page 290)
- Tea/herbal infusion of your choice

Day 23

Breakfast
- *Mint Chocolate Smoothie* (page 252)
- Organic coffee (optional: blended with 1–2 tablespoons of coconut oil, butter, or ghee) or tea/herbal infusion of your choice

Lunch
- Leftover *Italian Chicken and Eggplant Casserole* (page 268)
- Leftover *Roasted Cruciferous Vegetables* (page 290)
- Tea/herbal infusion of your choice

Snack (optional)
- *Butternut Squash Chips* (page 295)

Dinner
- 6 ounces of organic grass-fed lamb cooked in 1 tablespoon of coconut oil
- Steamed kale topped with 1 tablespoon of olive oil and seasoned to taste
- ½ cup of quinoa or rice cooked in bone broth (optional: sprinkle with turmeric and herbs)
- Tea/herbal infusion of your choice

Dessert
- *Cacao Blueberry Ice Cream* (page 302)

Day 24

Breakfast
- *Green Brain-Boosting Smoothie* (page 250)
- Organic coffee (optional: blended with 1–2 tablespoons of coconut oil, butter, or ghee) or tea/herbal infusion of your choice

Lunch
- *Creamy Tomato Soup* (page 261)
- ½ cup of fermented veggies
- ½ avocado
- Tea/herbal infusion of your choice

Snack (optional)
- Leftover *Butternut Squash Chips* (page 295)

Dinner
- *Roasted Salmon with Kefir, Garlic, and Avocado Sauce* (page 278)
- ½ cup of quinoa or rice cooked in bone broth (optional: sprinkle with turmeric and herbs)
- Side salad topped with homemade dressing: 1 tablespoon of olive oil mixed with apple cider vinegar and seasoned to taste
- Tea/herbal infusion of your choice

Day 25 (Optional Cleanse Day)

Breakfast

- *Cherry Vanilla Collagen Smoothie* (page 250)
- Organic coffee (optional: blended with 1–2 tablespoons of coconut oil, butter, or ghee) or tea/herbal infusion of your choice

Lunch

- *Pumpkin Pie Smoothie* (page 253)
- Tea/herbal infusion of your choice

Snack

- Spicy Heart Health Juice: ⅛ or less jalapeño, 1-inch knob ginger, 1 clove garlic, 1 medium raw beet, 2 carrots, 1 lemon, and 1 cucumber

Dinner

- Immune-Supporting Juice: 1 bell pepper (red, green, yellow, or orange), 1 small head broccoli (with stem), 1 lemon, 1 cucumber, 1-inch knob ginger, and 1 tablespoon apple cider vinegar
- *Strawberry Coconut Bone Broth Smoothie* (page 254)
- Tea/herbal infusion of your choice

Day 26

Breakfast

- *Black and Blue Berry Smoothie* (page 251)
- Organic coffee (optional: blended with
- 1–2 tablespoons of coconut oil, butter, or ghee) or tea/herbal infusion of your choice

Lunch

- Leftover *Creamy Tomato Soup* (page 261)
- *Cauliflower Tabbouleh Salad* (page 286)
- Tea/herbal infusion of your choice

Snack (optional)

- Raw veggies served with ½ cup hummus

Dinner

- *Chicken Thighs with Burst Tomatoes* (page 270)
- Steamed broccoli or brussels sprouts topped with 1 tablespoon of flax oil and seasoned to taste
- Tea/herbal infusion of your choice

Dessert

- *Almondy Chocolate Chip Cookies* (page 300)

Day 27

Breakfast

- *Loaded Kefir Breakfast Bowl* (page 256)

- Organic coffee (optional: blended with 1–2 tablespoons of coconut oil, butter, or ghee) or tea/herbal infusion of yourchoice

Lunch
- Leftover *Chicken Thighs with Burst Tomatoes* (page 270)
- Leftover *Cauliflower Tabbouleh Salad* (page 286) or ½ baked sweet potato
- Tea/herbal infusion of your choice

Snack (optional)
- 4 ounces of strawberries served with ½ cup full-fat cottage cheese

Dinner
- 2–3 eggs fried in 1 tablespoon of butter or avocado oil
- Sliced tomato and cucumber drizzled with lemon juice and olive oil and seasoned to taste
- Tea/herbal infusion of your choice

Day 28

Breakfast
- Omelet made with bell peppers, spinach, and tomatoes
- Organic coffee (optional: blended with 1–2 tablespoons of coconut oil, butter, or ghee) or tea/herbal infusion of your choice

Lunch

- 4 ounces of organic grass-fed beef cooked in 1 tablespoon of coconut oil
- Steamed or roasted asparagus drizzled with 1 tablespoon of olive oil and seasoned to taste
- ½ cup of brown rice cooked in bone broth and topped with turmeric and herbs of your choice

Snack (optional)

- *Almond Cacao Collagen Balls* (page 292)

Dinner

- 6 ounces of organic free-range chicken cooked in 1 tablespoon of coconut oil
- *Mashed Faux-tatoes* (page 289)
- ½ cup of fermented veggies

CHAPTER 13

The Collagen Diet Recipes

72 Delicious Options to Ensure You Get Enough Collagen

In this chapter, you'll find seventy-two of my favorite collagen recipes, from delicious smoothies that will help you start your day with a dose of long-lasting energy to simple (and yummy!) chicken, salmon, steak, and veggie meals you can whip up for dinner. I've also included some of my go-to snack items, such as Blueberry Macadamia Bars, and desserts, such as Banana Chia Pudding. They're proof that eating clean, healthful foods doesn't mean sacrificing decadent flavor. I can't wait for you to try them.

Some quick advice about which types of ingredients to choose:

■ Buy organic produce whenever you can. Organically grown fruits and veggies have the greatest health benefits and help you avoid pesticides and chemicals.

- When you're purchasing protein, opt for grass-fed beef, pasture-raised poultry and eggs, and wild-caught fish. These are the most nutritious options, and they don't contain hormones or other contaminants often found in conventionally raised animals.

- Buy full-fat versions of dairy products. They're far more nutritious than low-fat options, which are laden with sugar and missing the healthful fats your body needs to function its best.

It can feel overwhelming to try new recipes and novel ingredients, so I encourage you to approach these meals and snacks with a sense of curiosity, adventure, and fun. The best way to lose weight and improve your health is to enjoy the journey. My hope is that the delectable and nutritious options in this chapter will make it easy for you to do just that.

BREAKFASTS AND BEVERAGES

COLLAGEN COFFEE

SERVINGS: 1–2

TIME: 5 MINUTES

1½ cups organic brewed coffee

1 tablespoon butter from grass-fed cows

1 tablespoon coconut oil

1 scoop collagen protein

Place all ingredients in a high-powered blender and blend until smooth.

GOLDEN TEA

SERVINGS: 2

TIME: 5 MINUTES

1½ cups unsweetened almond milk

½ cup water

1 scoop turmeric bone broth protein

1 tablespoon ghee

1 tablespoon raw honey

Ground cinnamon or pumpkin pie spice to taste

In a small saucepan over medium-low heat, combine the almond milk, water, and bone broth protein.

Warm for 2 minutes.

Add the ghee and honey and stir for another 2 minutes.

Stir again and pour into glasses. Top with cinnamon or pumpkin pie spice (if using).

CHERRY VANILLA COLLAGEN SMOOTHIE

SERVINGS: 1
TIME: 5 MINUTES

1 cup unsweetened almond milk, plus more if needed

1 cup frozen cherries

1 scoop vanilla bone broth protein

3–4 ice cubes

Place all ingredients in a high-powered blender and blend until smooth, adding more almond milk as needed.

GREEN BRAIN-BOOSTING SMOOTHIE

SERVINGS: 1–2
TIME: 5 MINUTES

1/2 avocado

1/2 banana

1/2 cup fresh or frozen blueberries

1 scoop vanilla bone broth protein

6 whole shelled walnuts

1/2 cup water

Place all ingredients in a high-powered blender and blend until smooth.

BLACK AND BLUE BERRY SMOOTHIE

SERVINGS: 2
TIME: 5 MINUTES

1 cup frozen blueberries
1 cup frozen blackberries
½ frozen banana
1 cup unsweetened almond milk
½ cup full-fat unsweetened canned coconut milk
2 tablespoons almond butter

Place all ingredients in a high-powered blender and blend until smooth.

BLUEBERRY BLISS COLLAGEN SMOOTHIE

SERVINGS: 1–2
TIME: 5 MINUTES

1½ cups fresh or frozen blueberries
5 macadamia nuts
1 teaspoon vanilla extract
1 tablespoon raw honey or 2–3 drops liquid stevia (optional)
2 tablespoons collagen protein
2 cups full-fat unsweetened canned coconut milk, plus more if needed

Place all ingredients in a high-powered blender and blend until smooth, adding more coconut milk as needed.

CARROT GINGER BONE BROTH SHAKE

SERVINGS: 1–2
TIME: 5 MINUTES

3 cups grated carrots
1-inch knob fresh ginger, peeled and chopped
3 tablespoons bone broth protein
1¼ cups full-fat unsweetened canned coconut milk
1 tablespoon raw honey
Handful of ice cubes

Place all ingredients in a high-powered blender and blend until smooth.

MINT CHOCOLATE SMOOTHIE

SERVINGS: 1–2
TIME: 5 MINUTES

1½ cups unsweetened almond milk, plus more if needed
1–2 drops peppermint extract
2 tablespoons cacao powder
1 scoop chocolate bone broth protein
6 ice cubes, plus more if needed
Cacao nibs to taste

Place all ingredients except the cacao nibs in a high-powered blender and blend until smooth. Add more almond milk or ice as needed.

Top with cacao nibs.

PEACH PROBIOTIC SMOOTHIE

SERVINGS: 1–2
TIME: 5 MINUTES

1/2 banana

3/4 cup frozen peach chunks

1/2 cup full-fat unsweetened canned coconut milk or
full-fat plain goat-milk kefir or yogurt

1 1/2 cups unsweetened almond milk

1/2 teaspoon ground cinnamon

1 scoop vanilla bone broth protein

1/8 teaspoon vanilla extract

Place all ingredients in a high-powered blender and blend until smooth.

PUMPKIN PIE SMOOTHIE

SERVINGS: 1–2
TIME: 5 MINUTES

1/2 cup canned pumpkin puree

1/2 cup pureed cooked butternut squash

1/2 teaspoon pumpkin pie spice

1 1/2 cups unsweetened almond milk, plus more if needed

1 scoop vanilla bone broth protein

Place all ingredients in a high-powered blender and blend until smooth, adding more almond milk as needed.

STRAWBERRY COCONUT BONE BROTH SMOOTHIE

SERVINGS: 4

TIME: 5 MINUTES

¾ cup full-fat unsweetened canned coconut milk, plus
   more if needed

1 tablespoon vanilla bone broth protein

3 cups fresh or frozen strawberries

1 cup ice

Place all ingredients in a high-powered blender and blend until smooth, adding more coconut milk as needed.

ALMOND BERRY CEREAL

SERVINGS: 1

TIME: 5 MINUTES

½ cup full-fat unsweetened canned coconut milk

½ cup fresh or thawed frozen blueberries

¼ cup sliced almonds

¼ cup flaxseed meal

1 teaspoon ground cinnamon

Combine the coconut milk, blueberries, almonds, and flaxseed meal in a serving bowl. Sprinkle with cinnamon and enjoy.

COLLAGEN-ENHANCING VEGGIE-LOADED EGG BAKE

SERVINGS: 8
TIME: 40 MINUTES

8 large eggs
¼ cup unsweetened almond milk
1 teaspoon sea salt
2 scoops collagen protein (optional)
1 raw sweet potato, shredded
1 red bell pepper, diced
½ red onion, diced
1 cup chopped fresh spinach
½ cup cherry tomatoes, sliced
4–5 leaves basil, sliced

Preheat the oven to 375°F.

Whisk together the eggs, almond milk, salt, and collagen protein (if using) and set aside.

Place the shredded sweet potato in the bottom of a greased 9 × 13-inch casserole dish.

Pour the egg mixture over the sweet potato and evenly distribute the remaining vegetables over the top.

Bake for 25–30 minutes, or until the eggs are cooked through. Sprinkle with basil and serve.

LOADED KEFIR BREAKFAST BOWL

SERVINGS: 2
TIME: 5 MINUTES

2 cups full-fat plain goat-milk kefir
1 kiwifruit, sliced
1/2 cup fresh or frozen blueberries
1/2 cup fresh or frozen blackberries
1/4 cup goji berries
1/4 cup sliced almonds
1/4 cup chopped walnuts
3–4 drops liquid stevia per bowl (optional)

Combine all ingredients and divide between two bowls. Enjoy cold.

QUINOA PORRIDGE

SERVINGS: 1
TIME: 35 MINUTES

1/2 cup quinoa
1/4 teaspoon ground cinnamon
1 1/2 cups unsweetened almond milk
1/2 cup water
2 tablespoons raw honey
1 teaspoon vanilla extract
Pinch of sea salt

Combine the quinoa and cinnamon in a medium saucepan and place over medium heat. Cook, stirring frequently, for 3 minutes, or until quinoa is toasted.

Add the almond milk, water, honey, vanilla, and salt. Bring to a boil, then reduce heat and simmer for 25 minutes, stirring occasionally, until the porridge is thick and the grains are tender, adding more water if needed.

As the porridge cooks, stir more frequently to prevent burning, then transfer to a serving bowl and enjoy.

MAIN DISHES

BEEF AND BUTTERNUT SQUASH SOUP

SERVINGS: 6

TIME: 35 MINUTES

6 cups beef bone broth

1½ teaspoons ground ginger

1 teaspoon chipotle chili powder

1 teaspoon ground cumin

½ teaspoon sea salt

1 pound beef stew meat, sliced or cubed

1 yellow onion, diced

1 medium butternut squash, peeled and cubed

In a large pot over medium heat, bring the bone broth, spices, and salt to a simmer.

Add the remaining ingredients and return to a simmer. Reduce the heat to low and simmer for 25 minutes.

Serve warm.

BUTTERNUT BISQUE

SERVINGS: 4

TIME: I HOUR

4 tablespoons ghee

I red onion, chopped

I Granny Smith apple, peeled, cored, and chopped

2 teaspoons dried sage

I medium butternut squash, peeled and cut into chunks

4½ cups beef bone broth

I teaspoon ground nutmeg

Sea salt and black pepper to taste

In a large pot over medium heat, melt the ghee. Add the onion, apple, and sage and cook, stirring occasionally, for about 8 minutes.

Add the squash and bone broth. Bring to a simmer and cook for 15–20 minutes, or until the squash is fork-tender.

Using an immersion blender, blend the soup until the squash is pureed and the mixture is smooth. (Use caution when blending hot liquids.)

Heat through and season with the nutmeg, salt, and pepper before serving.

BUTTERNUT, CAULIFLOWER, AND CARROT SOUP

SERVINGS: 6–8

TIME: 1 HOUR

FOR THE ROASTED VEGGIES

2 cups chopped carrots

1 large butternut squash, peeled and chopped

1 small head cauliflower, chopped

1 onion, chopped

2 tablespoons avocado oil

Sea salt to taste

FOR THE BROTH

1 (15-ounce) can full-fat unsweetened coconut milk

3 cups bone broth or vegetable stock

2 tablespoons tahini

2 tablespoons curry powder

1-inch knob fresh ginger, peeled

1-inch piece fresh turmeric, peeled

1 teaspoon sea salt

1/2 teaspoon black pepper

FOR THE TOPPINGS

Coconut cream to taste

Raw or roasted pepitas to taste

Preheat the oven to 400°F.

On a large baking sheet, combine the veggies, avocado oil, and salt and stir to coat. Roast in the preheated oven for 45 minutes, or until fork-tender.

Place all the broth ingredients in a large bowl. Using an immersion blender, blend until smooth.

Once the veggies are roasted, carefully add them to the bowl with the broth ingredients. Set the immersion blender to the lowest setting and blend, slowly increasing the speed, until smooth.

Top with coconut cream and pepitas for a little crunch.

CHICKEN NOODLE SOUP

SERVINGS: 6–8

TIME: 1 HOUR

1 tablespoon avocado oil

1 cup diced yellow onion

1 cup diced carrots

1 cup diced celery

4 cups bone broth

4 cups water

3–4 cups shredded cooked chicken

2 bay leaves

Sea salt and black pepper to taste

1 teaspoon dried herbs, such as oregano, thyme, and parsley

16 ounces rice noodles, uncooked

Heat the avocado oil in a large pot over medium-high heat. Sauté the onion, carrots, and celery for 4–5 minutes, or until the vegetables soften and the onions are translucent.

Add the bone broth and water and bring to a low boil. Add the chicken and seasonings. Reduce the heat to low and simmer for 30 minutes, allowing the flavors to come together.

Add the noodles and simmer for 8–10 minutes, or until the noodles are fully cooked.

Discard the bay leaves and serve.

CREAMY TOMATO SOUP

SERVINGS: 6–8

TIME: 20 MINUTES

3 garlic cloves, pressed or minced
1 tablespoon coconut oil
4 cups diced fresh tomatoes
1¾ cups full-fat unsweetened canned coconut milk
½ teaspoon sea salt
2 teaspoons apple cider vinegar
4 cups beef bone broth
4 scoops collagen protein
Minced fresh basil to taste
Black pepper to taste

In a medium pot over medium-low heat, sauté the garlic in the coconut oil for 5 minutes, or until lightly browned.

In a high-powered blender, puree the tomatoes, coconut milk, salt, vinegar, bone broth, and collagen protein until well combined.

Pour the mixture into the pot with the garlic and bring to a simmer, stirring occasionally.

Simmer for 10–15 minutes. Remove from the heat and allow the soup to rest for 5 minutes.

Serve topped with the fresh basil and pepper.

SLOW COOKER GINGERED BEEF AND BROCCOLI SOUP

SERVINGS: 4

TIME: 8 HOURS

2 teaspoons coconut oil

¼ cup coconut aminos (a liquid made from the aged sap of coconut blossoms that serves as a low-glycemic, vegan, gluten-free alternative to soy sauce)

2 tablespoons apple cider vinegar

2 garlic cloves, smashed

½ teaspoon crushed red pepper flakes

1 tablespoon grated fresh ginger

1 pound rib-eye steak, sliced into strips

2 cups beef bone broth

2 scoops collagen protein

1 head broccoli, cut into 1-inch pieces

1 tablespoon sesame seeds

In a slow cooker, combine the coconut oil, coconut aminos, vinegar, garlic, red pepper flakes, and ginger.

Place the steak in the slow cooker and flip to coat.

In a small bowl, combine the bone broth and collagen protein. Stir until combined and pour into the slow cooker.

Cook on low for 6–8 hours.

Add the broccoli 1 hour before serving.

Sprinkle the sesame seeds over the top and serve.

INDIAN CURRY SOUP

SERVINGS: 4

TIME: 35 MINUTES

6 cups beef bone broth

1 tablespoon grated fresh ginger

3 tablespoons curry powder

1 yellow onion, chopped

2 cups chopped cauliflower florets

2 red bell peppers, chopped

1 teaspoon cayenne pepper

1¾ cups full-fat unsweetened canned coconut milk

In a large pot over medium heat, bring the bone broth and ginger to a simmer. Add the curry powder, onion, cauliflower, red peppers, and cayenne.

Bring to a boil, then reduce the heat to medium-low and simmer for 15 minutes.

Add the coconut milk and stir until well combined. Cook for an additional 5–10 minutes.

Allow the soup to rest for 5 minutes before serving.

MEATBALL SOUP

SERVINGS: 4–6
TIME: 50 MINUTES

1½ pounds ground bison or beef
2 large eggs, whisked
1½ teaspoons sea salt, divided
1 teaspoon smoked paprika or cayenne pepper
2 tablespoons coconut oil
6 cups beef bone broth
2 bay leaves
4 carrots, chopped
1 large sweet potato, chopped
1 cup fresh or frozen cut green beans
1 cup fresh peas
2 fresh tomatoes, chopped

In a medium bowl, mix together the meat, eggs, ½ teaspoon salt, and paprika or cayenne. Roll into small meatballs.

In a large pot over medium heat, heat the oil. Add the meatballs and cook for 5-8 minutes, flipping halfway through.

Add the bone broth, remaining salt, bay leaves, carrots, and sweet potato. Bring the soup to a simmer over medium-high heat.

Add the remaining ingredients and simmer for 20 minutes, or until the sweet potato is tender. Discard the bay leaves and serve immediately.

"NOODLE" BOWLS

SERVINGS: 4

TIME: 50 MINUTES

3 boneless skinless chicken breasts

2 tablespoons coconut oil, melted and divided

1 tablespoon sea salt, plus more to taste

1 tablespoon black pepper, plus more to taste

1/2 medium red onion, diced

3 stalks celery, chopped

6 carrots, chopped

4 cups chopped kale, stems removed

8 cups beef bone broth

3 medium zucchini, spiralized into noodles

Chopped fresh basil to taste

Preheat the oven to 325°F.

Line a baking sheet with parchment paper. Place the chicken on the paper, drizzle with 1 tablespoon of the coconut oil, and sprinkle with 1 tablespoon of the salt and 1 tablespoon of the pepper. Bake for 30 minutes, or until the internal temperature of the chicken reaches 165°F.

In a large stockpot over medium heat, combine the remaining coconut oil, onion, celery, and carrots and cook for 8–10 minutes.

Add the kale and bone broth. Stir to combine.

Reduce the heat to low and let simmer for 25 minutes.

Take the chicken out of the oven and allow to cool for 5 minutes.

Using two forks, shred the chicken and add it to the stockpot. Simmer for another 15 minutes.

Add the spiralized zucchini, stirring to combine.

Add salt and pepper to taste and serve topped with the fresh basil.

WHITE BEAN AND KALE SOUP

SERVINGS: 2

TIME: 40 MINUTES

1 quart organic free-range chicken broth, divided

4 links pork-free chicken sausage

1/2 onion, chopped

Sea salt and black pepper to taste

4 cups cooked white beans, such as cannellini, navy, or
     great northern, divided

1/2 bunch kale, stems removed and leaves roughly
     chopped

1 tablespoon butter from grass-fed cows

In a large pot, heat 1/4 cup of the broth over medium heat.

Slice the chicken sausage into bite-size pieces and add to the pot. Cook, stirring occasionally, for 10 minutes.

Add the onion, salt, and pepper and cook another 10 minutes.

Meanwhile, place 2 cups of the beans and 1 cup of the broth in a blender. Blend until smooth, then set aside.

Add the remaining broth to the pot and bring to a boil. Add the kale, then cover, reduce heat, and simmer, stirring occasionally, for 5 minutes.

Uncover, then add the remaining beans, bean puree, and butter. Season to taste, then simmer until heated through. Serve immediately.

WILD RICE AND SPINACH SOUP

SERVINGS: 2
TIME: 45 MINUTES

1 tablespoon butter from grass-fed cows
1 cup wild rice, cooked
1 onion, chopped
1 red bell pepper, chopped
1 quart organic free-range chicken broth
1/2 cup chopped carrots
7 ounces baby spinach leaves, coarsely chopped
1/4 teaspoon sea salt
Black pepper to taste

Melt the butter in a large saucepan over medium heat. Add the rice, onion, and bell pepper. Cook for 3 minutes, or until the vegetables soften and the rice is heated through.

Stir in the broth and cook for 7 minutes, or until the mixture begins to boil.

Cover, reduce the heat to low, and simmer for 15 minutes, stirring occasionally.

Add the carrots, cover, and cook for 10 minutes, or until the carrots are tender.

Add the spinach, salt, and pepper and cook for 2 minutes, or until the spinach is wilted. Serve immediately.

ITALIAN CHICKEN AND EGGPLANT CASSEROLE

SERVINGS: 4

TIME: 50 MINUTES

1 pound boneless skinless chicken breasts

1 large eggplant

½ cup almond meal

1 tablespoon Italian seasoning

1 teaspoon sea salt

2 large eggs

24 ounces prepared marinara sauce with no sugar added

1 cup shredded whole-milk mozzarella cheese

1 bunch fresh basil, sliced

Preheat the oven to 375°F.

Slice the chicken breasts horizontally into two thin cutlets. Slice the eggplant into ¼-inch-thick slices. Pat the chicken and eggplant dry with paper towels.

In a small bowl, mix the almond meal, Italian seasoning, and salt. In a separate bowl, whisk the eggs.

Dip the eggplant and chicken slices in the egg, then in the almond meal mixture. Arrange the pieces in a 9 × 13-inch casserole dish.

Top with marinara sauce and cheese. Bake for 30–35 minutes, or until the internal temperature of the chicken reaches 165°F.

Top with the basil and enjoy.

CHICKEN TENDERS

SERVINGS: 4
TIME: 20 MINUTES

2 large eggs
1 scoop collagen protein
Italian seasoning to taste
Sea salt to taste
4 boneless skinless chicken breasts, sliced into strips
1 cup brown rice flour or coconut flour
1 tablespoon coconut oil

In a medium bowl, beat the eggs slightly. Add the collagen protein, Italian seasoning, and salt, mixing well.

Dip the strips of chicken in the egg mixture, then coat with the flour.

In a medium frying pan over medium heat, melt the coconut oil. Fry the chicken, turning once, until golden brown and the internal temperature of the chicken reaches 165°F. Serve warm.

CHICKEN THIGHS WITH BURST TOMATOES

SERVINGS: 2

TIME: 40 MINUTES

2 bone-in skin-on chicken thighs
1 tablespoon sea salt
1 teaspoon black pepper
1 cup fresh cherry tomatoes
2 sprigs thyme
2 tablespoons red wine vinegar

Pat the chicken thighs dry and season with the salt and pepper.

Arrange the chicken skin side down in a cold skillet. Place the skillet over medium heat and, once hot, cook for 10–12 minutes without turning. Once the skin is browned, remove the chicken from the skillet and set aside.

Add the tomatoes, thyme, and red wine vinegar to the skillet. Cook for about 10 minutes, stirring occasionally, until most of the tomatoes have burst on their own. Reduce the heat to medium-low.

Return the chicken to the pan with the tomatoes, this time skin side up. Cook another 10 minutes, or until the internal temperature of the chicken reaches 165°F.

ROASTED CHICKEN WITH ROMA TOMATOES AND ONIONS

SERVINGS: 4

TIME: 40 MINUTES

2 teaspoons coconut oil

2 pounds bone-in skin-on chicken thighs

2 tablespoons ghee

2 tablespoons minced garlic

½ teaspoon sea salt

½ teaspoon black pepper

½ white onion, sliced

1 cup sliced Roma tomatoes

½ cup chicken bone broth

Chopped fresh basil to taste

Preheat the oven to 425°F.

In a skillet over medium-high heat, heat the coconut oil.

Pat the chicken thighs with a paper towel to remove excess moisture. In a bowl, mix together the ghee, garlic, salt, and pepper and spread the mixture under the skin of the chicken and on the outside.

Place the chicken thighs in the skillet skin side down and sear for 5 minutes, or until browned.

Flip the chicken over and add the sliced onion and tomatoes.

Pour the bone broth around the chicken.

Place the skillet in the oven and roast for 15–20 minutes, or until the chicken reaches an internal temperature of 165°F.

Let cool for 5 minutes and top with the basil before serving.

SPAGHETTI SQUASH WITH ROASTED CHICKEN, LEMON, AND PARSLEY

SERVINGS: 4

TIME: 1 HOUR

1 medium spaghetti squash

2 tablespoons ghee, divided

1½ pounds bone-in skin-on chicken thighs

¼ teaspoon sea salt

¼ teaspoon black pepper

2 tablespoons chopped garlic

Juice of 1 lemon

½ cup chicken bone broth

1 scoop collagen protein

¼ cup chopped parsley, divided

Preheat the oven to 425°F.

Cut the spaghetti squash in half and scoop out the seeds. Place the squash facedown on a baking sheet and bake for 40–50 minutes, or until soft.

Let cool, then use a fork to scrape the flesh out. Set aside.

In a large skillet over medium-high heat, heat 1 tablespoon of the ghee. Season the chicken with the salt and pepper.

Place the chicken in the pan skin side down. Sear for 5 minutes, then remove the chicken from the pan and set aside.

Add the garlic to the skillet and brown for about 30 seconds. Add the lemon juice, broth, collagen protein, and 1 tablespoon of the parsley and stir.

Return the chicken to the pan, skin side up. Place the pan in the oven and roast for 10–12 minutes, or until the internal temperature of the chicken reaches 165°F.

Toss the hot spaghetti squash with the remaining ghee. Divide the spaghetti squash among four serving plates, top with the chicken and remaining parsley, and serve.

ZUCCHINI AND CHICKEN SALAD

SERVINGS: 1–2
TIME: 15 MINUTES

¼ cup extra virgin olive oil
¼ cup freshly squeezed lemon juice
Sea salt and black pepper to taste
1¼ pounds zucchini, thinly sliced
1 tablespoon grapeseed oil
1 pound boneless skinless chicken breasts
8 ounces baby spinach leaves, chopped
½ red onion, thinly sliced
¾ cup chopped pecans
¼ cup chopped fresh mint

In a large bowl, whisk together the olive oil, lemon juice, salt, and pepper. Add the zucchini and toss to coat. Set aside.

Heat the grapeseed oil in a skillet over medium heat. Add the chicken and season with the salt and pepper.

Cook for 7 minutes on each side, or until golden brown. Remove from the skillet and slice into thin strips.

In a serving bowl, toss the chicken with the zucchini mixture, spinach, onion, pecans, and mint. Serve immediately.

CURRIED TURKEY SALAD

SERVINGS: 4
TIME: 5 MINUTES

4 turkey breasts, cooked and diced
1 stalk celery, diced
4 scallions, white and tender green parts only, chopped
1 Granny Smith apple, peeled, cored, and chopped
⅔ cup golden raisins
½ cup chopped pecans
⅛ teaspoon black pepper
½ teaspoon curry powder
¾ cup vegan mayonnaise made with grapeseed oil, such as Vegenaise

Combine all ingredients in a large bowl and mix well.

Distribute among four serving bowls and serve immediately.

QUINOA-STUFFED BELL PEPPERS

SERVINGS: 2–4

TIME: 45 MINUTES

6 cups water

2 cups quinoa, rinsed and drained

2 scoops bone broth protein

2 bell peppers (any color), halved and seeded

Sea salt and black pepper to taste

1 teaspoon coconut oil

1 onion, diced

1 zucchini, chopped

2 tablespoons minced garlic

1 tablespoon Italian seasoning

½ cup chopped parsley

1 cup crumbled goat cheese

Preheat the oven to 450°F.

In a medium pot, combine the water, quinoa, and bone broth protein. Cook quinoa according to package directions.

Meanwhile, sprinkle the bell peppers with the salt and pepper. Place the peppers on a baking sheet and roast cut side down for 20 minutes, or until the skin begins to char. Remove from the oven and reduce the oven temperature to 375°F.

While the bell peppers roast, melt the oil in a skillet over medium heat. Add the onion, zucchini, garlic, and Italian seasoning. Season with additional salt and pepper. Cook, stirring occasionally, for 10–12 minutes, or until the vegetables are tender. Add the quinoa to the skillet. Sprinkle with the parsley and stir to combine.

When the bell peppers are ready, turn them cut side up and fill the halves evenly with the quinoa mixture. Heat in the oven until warmed through. Top with the cheese and serve.

SPICY WALNUT TACOS

SERVINGS: 2–3
TIME: 10 MINUTES

1½ cups ground raw walnuts
1½ teaspoons ground cumin
¾ teaspoon ground coriander
2 teaspoons coconut aminos (see page 262)
Pinch of cayenne pepper
Bibb lettuce leaves
Prepared salsa to taste
Prepared guacamole to taste

In a food processor, combine the walnuts, cumin, coriander, coconut aminos, and cayenne pepper. Process until a coarse mixture forms.

Spoon an equal portion of the mixture onto each lettuce leaf. Top with salsa and guacamole and serve.

LEAFY GREEN SALAD WITH SALMON

SERVINGS: 1

TIME: 10 MINUTES

FOR THE DRESSING

2 tablespoons extra virgin olive oil

2 tablespoons white balsamic vinegar

1 teaspoon Dijon mustard

½ teaspoon maple syrup or monk fruit syrup (optional)

FOR THE SALAD

2 cups torn leafy greens, such as spinach, kale, or baby chard

¼ cup fresh blueberries

2 tablespoons mixed raw nuts, such as almonds, walnuts, and cashews

1–2 tablespoons mixed raw seeds, such as pepitas, sunflower seeds, and flaxseeds

2 tablespoons crumbled goat cheese

½ ripe avocado, sliced

1 fillet (6 ounces) wild-caught salmon, roasted*

In a small bowl, whisk together the dressing ingredients.

In a large bowl, assemble the salad ingredients. Drizzle with the desired amount of dressing and enjoy.

---

* For roasting instructions, see the Roasted Salmon with Kefir, Garlic, and Avocado Sauce recipe on the next page.

ROASTED SALMON WITH KEFIR, GARLIC, AND AVOCADO SAUCE

SERVINGS: 4

TIME: 45 MINUTES

FOR THE FISH

1½ pounds wild-caught salmon fillets

2 tablespoons extra virgin olive oil

½ teaspoon sea salt

½–1 teaspoon black pepper

2 tablespoons freshly squeezed lemon juice

FOR THE SAUCE

1 ripe avocado

2 cups full-fat plain goat-milk kefir, or more if needed

2 scoops collagen protein

2 garlic cloves, smashed

¼–½ teaspoon sea salt

Preheat the oven to 425°F. Line a baking sheet with parchment paper.

Rub the salmon with the olive oil, season with the salt and pepper, and place it skin side down on the prepared baking sheet. Drizzle with the lemon juice and roast for 15 minutes, or until the salmon flakes when gently pressed.

Meanwhile, in a high-powered blender, combine the sauce ingredients and blend on high speed until well combined. Add more kefir as needed.

Remove the salmon from the oven. Peel the skin off and break the flesh into chunks. Arrange on serving plates and drizzle with the sauce. Serve immediately.

STIR-FRY SALMON

SERVINGS: 2

TIME: 20 MINUTES

¼ cup coconut aminos (see page 262)

2 teaspoons rice vinegar

2 teaspoons sesame oil

1 cup chopped bell peppers (any color)

1 onion, chopped

1 pound wild-caught salmon, skinned and cut into 1½-inch cubes

1 tablespoon coconut oil

1 tablespoon finely chopped fresh ginger

1 tablespoon sesame seeds

4 garlic cloves, finely chopped

1½ cups chopped fresh mushrooms

1 head broccoli, chopped and blanched

In a large skillet over medium heat, combine the coconut aminos, vinegar, sesame oil, bell peppers, and onion. Cook the peppers and onion until translucent.

Add the salmon and coat with the mixture.

Add the coconut oil, ginger, sesame seeds, garlic, mushrooms, and broccoli and stir.

Continue to cook, stirring occasionally, for 10 minutes, or until the salmon is cooked through. Serve warm.

SEARED TUNA WITH ASPARAGUS

SERVINGS: 2

TIME: 25 MINUTES

2 wild-caught tuna fillets (6 ounces each)

¼ cup coconut aminos (see page 262)

Juice of ½ lime

1 bunch asparagus

2 tablespoons avocado oil, divided

½ teaspoon sea salt

2 teaspoons toasted sesame seeds

Preheat the broiler.

In a medium nonreactive bowl, marinate the tuna in the coconut aminos and lime juice for 15 minutes.

Place the asparagus on a baking pan and toss with 1 tablespoon of the avocado oil and the salt. Place under the broiler for 6–8 minutes, or until the asparagus has softened and is a little browned.

Heat the remaining avocado oil in a large skillet over medium-high heat. Add the marinated tuna fillets and cook for 2 minutes. Flip the fish and cook for another 2 minutes. If desired, cook the sides of the fillets for 1 minute each.

Arrange the tuna on serving plates and sprinkle with the sesame seeds. Slice and serve with the asparagus.

GRILLED FLAT IRON STEAK

SERVINGS: 4–5
TIME: 40 MINUTES

1½ pounds flat iron steak
¼ cup coconut aminos (see page 262)
Juice of 1 lime
1 teaspoon sea salt
1 tablespoon extra virgin olive oil

In a medium nonreactive bowl, marinate the steak in the coconut aminos, lime juice, and salt for 30 minutes.

Grease an outdoor grill or a stovetop grill pan with the olive oil and heat over medium-high heat.

Place the steak on the grill or grill pan and cook for 4–5 minutes on each side, or until the meat is done to your liking.

Let the steak rest on a cutting board for 10 minutes. Slice it into ¼–½-inch-thick slices and enjoy.

SHEPHERD'S PIE

SERVINGS: 8–10
TIME: 1¼ HOURS

FOR THE FILLING

2 tablespoons coconut oil
1 pound ground beef or lamb
2 large carrots, sliced thin
1 yellow onion, diced
1½ cups frozen green peas, thawed

FOR THE GRAVY

1 scoop bone broth protein

2 cups water or beef or lamb stock

1 cup chopped cauliflower

1 onion, chopped

½ teaspoon sea salt

½ teaspoon black pepper

2 teaspoons minced fresh thyme

2 teaspoons minced fresh rosemary

3 garlic cloves, pressed or minced

1½ teaspoons Worcestershire sauce

4 tablespoons butter from grass-fed cows, at room
    temperature

½ cup arrowroot starch

FOR THE TOPPING

1 recipe Mashed Faux-tatoes (page 289)

To make the filling, heat the coconut oil in a large skillet over medium-high heat. Add the meat, carrots, and onion. Cook, stirring often, until the meat is browned and the vegetables have begun to soften, 10–15 minutes.

Drain the fat from the skillet, then add the peas and stir to combine. Transfer the filling to the bottom of an 8 × 8-inch baking dish and set aside.

Preheat the oven to 400°F.

To make the gravy, combine the bone broth protein, water or stock, cauliflower, onion, salt, and pepper in a medium pot. Heat, uncovered, over medium-high heat until simmering. Lower the heat and simmer for 10 minutes. Stir in the thyme, rosemary, and garlic and remove from the heat.

In a high-powered blender, combine the Worcestershire sauce and butter. Pour in the stock mixture and blend until smooth. Add the arrowroot starch and blend until smooth. Pour the gravy evenly over the filling in the dish.

Prepare the Mashed Faux-tatoes according to the recipe directions and spread on top of the meat and vegetables.

Bake in the preheated oven for 30 minutes, or until the topping begins to brown and the gravy is bubbling. Cool for 10 minutes before serving.

SLOW COOKER STEAK FAJITAS

SERVINGS: 6–8
TIME: 8 HOURS

FOR THE FAJITAS

1½ pounds skirt steak
1 green bell pepper, sliced
1 red bell pepper, sliced
1 red onion, sliced
1–2 jalapeños, seeded, deveined, and sliced
1–2 cups prepared salsa
1 tablespoon chili powder
1 tablespoon dried oregano
1 tablespoon ground cumin
1 tablespoon garlic powder
½ tablespoon onion powder
1 teaspoon smoked paprika
1 teaspoon sea salt
1 teaspoon black pepper
6–8 almond-flour tortillas

FOR THE TOPPINGS

Plain goat-milk yogurt
Chopped fresh tomatoes
Chopped scallions
Fresh cilantro leaves

Place all the fajita ingredients except the tortillas in a slow cooker and cook on low for 8 hours.

Serve on the tortillas and top as desired with the yogurt, tomatoes, scallions, and cilantro.

SIDES

BEAN SALAD

SERVINGS: 8–10
TIME: 10 MINUTES

FOR THE DRESSING

¼ cup extra virgin olive oil
¼ cup freshly squeezed lime juice
2 garlic cloves, minced
1 tablespoon Dijon mustard
1 teaspoon maple syrup (optional)

FOR THE SALAD

1 (15-ounce) can garbanzo beans
1 (15-ounce) can great northern beans
1 (15-ounce) can kidney beans
½ red onion, diced
2 celery stalks, diced
1 cup chopped cilantro
1 teaspoon sea salt

In a small bowl, whisk together the dressing ingredients and set aside.

Drain and rinse the beans. Combine with the remaining salad ingredients in a large bowl.

Drizzle with the dressing and toss. Serve chilled.

CAULIFLOWER TABBOULEH SALAD

SERVINGS: 6
TIME: 35 MINUTES

1 large head cauliflower, chopped
½ cup freshly squeezed lemon juice
¾ cup extra virgin olive oil
1 bunch parsley, leaves and tender stems only, chopped
1 bunch scallions, white and tender green parts only,
    chopped
2 cups chopped Roma tomatoes
1 teaspoon sea salt, or more to taste
1 teaspoon black pepper, or more to taste

Place the chopped cauliflower in a food processor and process until the pieces resemble grains of rice.

In a large nonreactive bowl, combine the processed cauliflower and the lemon juice.

Add the olive oil, parsley, scallions, tomatoes, salt, and pepper. Stir thoroughly.

Taste and add more salt and pepper if needed.

Cover and refrigerate for at least 4 hours, stirring every hour.

CREAMED SPINACH

SERVINGS: 6

TIME: 20 MINUTES

2 tablespoons butter from grass-fed cows

2 garlic cloves, minced

1/2 yellow onion, finely diced

1 (10-ounce) package frozen spinach, thawed and well drained

1/4 cup heavy cream

1/2 cup shredded whole-milk mozzarella cheese

1/2 cup shredded Parmesan cheese

In a large saucepan over medium heat, melt the butter. Add the garlic and onion and cook for 4–5 minutes, or until the onion is translucent.

Add the spinach and cook for another 3–4 minutes.

Stir in the heavy cream and cheeses. Cook on low, stirring often, for 7–9 minutes, or until the cheese has melted and the sauce has thickened. Serve warm.

LEMON PEPPER GREEN BEANS

SERVINGS: 8
TIME: 10 MINUTES

2 tablespoons coconut oil
3 pounds fresh green beans, trimmed
2 garlic cloves, minced
1/4 cup freshly squeezed lemon juice
2 teaspoons grated lemon zest
Sea salt and black pepper to taste

Heat the oil in a large skillet over medium heat. Add the green beans and garlic and stir-fry for 3 minutes, or until the beans are crisp-tender.

Reduce the heat, then add the lemon juice, zest, salt, and pepper.

Cover and steam for 2–3 minutes, stirring occasionally. Serve immediately.

MAPLE-GLAZED ROSEMARY CARROTS

SERVINGS: 4–6
TIME: 25 MINUTES

3 cups sliced carrots
2 tablespoons coconut oil
2 tablespoons maple syrup
1 1/2 tablespoons chopped fresh rosemary
1/2 teaspoon sea salt
1/2 teaspoon black pepper

Place the carrots in a medium skillet and add just enough water to cover. Bring to a boil, then reduce the heat and simmer for 5–10 minutes, or until the water has evaporated and the carrots are soft.

Reduce the heat to low, stir in the remaining ingredients, and cook for another 5–10 minutes.

Serve immediately.

MASHED FAUX-TATOES

SERVINGS: 4
TIME: 25 MINUTES

1 medium head cauliflower, cut into chunks
2 scoops collagen protein
4 tablespoons ghee
½ teaspoon sea salt
½ teaspoon black pepper
Chopped fresh parsley to taste

In a large pot fitted with a steamer basket, steam the cauliflower for 10 minutes, or until the florets are tender.

Combine the cauliflower, collagen protein, ghee, salt, and pepper in a food processor. Process until smooth.

Top with the parsley and serve immediately.

MASHED SWEET POTATOES

SERVINGS: 2–4
TIME: 25 MINUTES

2 sweet potatoes, chopped
½ cup full-fat unsweetened canned coconut milk or
    heavy cream
2 tablespoons ghee or coconut oil
1 teaspoon sea salt
2 scoops collagen protein (optional)
½ cup shredded unsweetened coconut (optional)

Bring a pot of water to a boil, add the potatoes, and boil for 15 minutes, or until fork-tender.

Drain the potatoes and return them to the pot. Add the coconut milk, ghee or coconut oil, salt, and collagen protein (if using). Mash with a masher or a fork and stir everything together until the ingredients are evenly incorporated.

Stir in the shredded coconut (if using) and serve warm.

ROASTED CRUCIFEROUS VEGETABLES

SERVINGS: 4
TIME: 30 MINUTES

1 cup broccoli florets
1 cup cauliflower florets
1 cup quartered brussels sprouts
2 tablespoons avocado oil
1 teaspoon garlic powder
1 teaspoon sea salt

Preheat the oven to 425°F.

Combine all ingredients in a large bowl, then spread the mixture out onto a large baking sheet.

Bake for 20–25 minutes, tossing halfway through, until the vegetables are browned and crispy. Serve warm.

SWEET POTATO FRIES

SERVINGS: 3–6
TIME: I HOUR

1–1½ pounds sweet potatoes
¼ cup coconut oil, melted
½ teaspoon sea salt
½ teaspoon paprika
¼ teaspoon ground cinnamon

Preheat the oven to 425°F. Peel the potatoes and cut lengthwise into ½-inch-wide strips.

Place the potatoes along with the remaining ingredients in a resealable plastic bag and shake until the potatoes are completely coated. Spread onto a baking sheet.

Cook for 30–45 minutes, tossing every 10 minutes.

Transfer to a paper-towel-lined plate and serve warm.

SNACKS

ALMOND CACAO COLLAGEN BALLS

YIELD: 8–10 BALLS

TIME: 20 MINUTES

½ cup raw almonds

½ cup almond flour

3 tablespoons coconut butter

3 tablespoons almond butter

2 tablespoons maple syrup

2 tablespoons unsweetened almond milk, plus more if needed

2 scoops collagen protein (optional)

Handful of cacao nibs

In a food processor, combine the almonds, almond flour, coconut butter, almond butter, maple syrup, almond milk, and collagen protein (if using).

Process until the mixture is smooth and doughy. You may need 1 extra teaspoon or so of almond milk, depending on how dry the mixture is.

Transfer to a mixing bowl, add the cacao nibs, and mix with your hands or a spoon.

Using your hands, roll the dough into bite-size balls.

Freeze for 10–15 minutes, or until firm. Store in an airtight container in the refrigerator.

BLUEBERRY MACADAMIA BARS

SERVINGS: 6

TIME: 2¼ HOURS

½ cup melted coconut butter

¼ cup raw honey

1 teaspoon vanilla extract

Pinch of sea salt

4 scoops vanilla bone broth protein

½ cup dried blueberries

½ cup chopped raw macadamia nuts

3 tablespoons water

In a medium bowl, whisk together the coconut butter, honey, vanilla, and salt. Add the bone broth protein and stir well. Add the remaining ingredients and combine thoroughly.

Pour into a greased loaf pan. Refrigerate for 1–2 hours, then cut into bars.

BLUEBERRY MUFFINS

SERVINGS: 12
TIME: 40 MINUTES

2 tablespoons coconut oil, melted, plus more for
    greasing pan
1 cup oat flour
1/2 cup almond flour
1/2 teaspoon baking powder
1/4 teaspoon sea salt
6 scoops collagen protein
3 large eggs
1/2 cup raw honey
1/2 cup unsweetened applesauce
1 teaspoon vanilla extract
1 teaspoon apple cider vinegar
1 cup fresh or frozen blueberries

Preheat the oven to 350°F.

Grease a standard muffin tin with coconut oil and set aside.

In a large mixing bowl, whisk together the oat flour, almond flour, baking powder, salt, and collagen protein.

In a separate bowl, combine the eggs, honey, applesauce, vanilla, vinegar, and 2 tablespoons melted coconut oil. Stir until well combined.

Slowly add the dry mixture to the wet mixture and stir well.

Fold the blueberries into the batter.

Fill each compartment 3/4 full, then bake for 30 minutes, or until golden brown on top.

BUTTERNUT SQUASH CHIPS

SERVINGS: 4–6

TIME: 40 MINUTES

1 large butternut squash
1 tablespoon avocado oil
2 teaspoons dried sage
1 teaspoon sea salt

Preheat the oven to 450°F. Line a baking sheet with foil.

Peel the butternut squash. Use a mandoline or a sharp knife to cut it into thin rounds. Cut until you reach the seeded part of the squash. You may either remove the seeds and cut more slices or reserve the rest of the squash for another use.

Arrange the squash slices on the prepared baking sheet and drizzle with the avocado oil. Sprinkle the sage and salt evenly across the squash.

Bake for 15 minutes. Flip the chips and bake for another 7–9 minutes, or until crispy.

CHOCOLATE CHERRY PROTEIN BARS

SERVINGS: 4–6
TIME: 1½ HOURS

1 cup dried cherries
5 pitted Medjool dates
1 cup cashew butter
½ cup cacao powder
3 tablespoons collagen protein
1 tablespoon flaxseeds
2 tablespoons coconut oil
½ teaspoon sea salt

Line an 8 × 8-inch baking dish with parchment paper.

In a food processor, combine the dried cherries and dates and pulse into small pieces.

Add the remaining ingredients and pulse until a dough forms.

Spread the dough out evenly in the baking dish.

Place the dough in the freezer for 1 hour.

Cut into squares and store in an airtight container in the freezer.

CUCUMBER SALSA

SERVINGS: 2–4

TIME: 5 MINUTES

3 cups quartered cherry tomatoes

1 cup chopped green, red, and yellow bell peppers

2 medium cucumbers, peeled, seeded, and chopped

1 jalapeño, seeded, deveined, and chopped

1 small Vidalia onion

1 garlic clove, minced

¼ cup freshly squeezed lime juice

1 teaspoon minced fresh parsley

Combine all ingredients in a large bowl and serve.

GUACAMOLE

SERVINGS: 8–10

TIME: 10 MINUTES

4 ripe avocados

½ red onion, finely diced

¼ cup chopped cilantro

2 garlic cloves, minced

1 tablespoon chili powder

1 tablespoon ground cumin

1 teaspoon sea salt

Juice of 1 lime

1 small jalapeño, seeded, deveined, and finely diced
    (optional)

1 scoop collagen protein (optional)

Remove the avocado flesh from the skins. Save one seed and discard the rest. Mash the avocado in a large bowl with a fork.

Stir in the remaining ingredients until everything is well incorporated. Place the saved seed in the middle of the bowl. This helps keep the guacamole from browning.

Allow the guacamole to sit for 10 minutes so the flavors can meld. Remove the seed, stir, and serve.

NO-BAKE BONE BROTH PROTEIN MUFFINS

SERVINGS: 12

TIME: 1¼ HOURS

4 cups cashews

3 cups pitted Medjool dates

2 tablespoons cashew butter

2 teaspoons vanilla extract

2 teaspoons ground cinnamon

4 tablespoons vanilla bone broth protein

2 tablespoons water

⅛ teaspoon sea salt

In a food processor, pulse the cashews until small chunks form. Add the remaining ingredients and process on high speed until a dough forms, scraping the sides as needed.

Place liners in a muffin tin or cupcake pan. Evenly distribute the dough in each compartment of the pan.

Cover and freeze for 1 hour before serving.

SPICED NUTS

SERVINGS: 2
TIME: 10 MINUTES

½ cup raw honey

2 cups pecan halves, whole almonds, or walnut halves

1 teaspoon ground cinnamon

¼ teaspoon cayenne pepper

Preheat the oven to 300°F.

In a medium bowl, combine all ingredients and toss until the nuts are completely coated.

Spread the nuts onto a cookie sheet in a single layer. Toast for 5 minutes, or until the nuts are fragrant, tossing occasionally.

Serve immediately or let cool and store in an airtight container.

DESSERTS

ALMONDY CHOCOLATE CHIP COOKIES

SERVINGS: 12–14

TIME: 20 MINUTES

2 cups almond flour

½ teaspoon baking soda

½ teaspoon sea salt

¼ cup maple syrup

1 tablespoon plus 1 teaspoon coconut oil, melted

1 teaspoon vanilla extract

¼ cup stevia-sweetened or unsweetened chocolate
  chips

2 scoops collagen protein (optional)

Preheat the oven to 350°F. Line a baking sheet with parchment paper.

Combine all the ingredients in a medium bowl.

Divide dough into 12–14 portions and roll into balls. Place on the prepared baking sheet about 2 inches apart.

Press down each cookie with a fork. Bake for 10–12 minutes, or until the edges are golden.

APPLE CRISP

SERVINGS: 8

TIME: 10 MINUTES

8 Granny Smith apples, cored

1 cup raisins, soaked in hot water for 15 minutes and
   drained

2 teaspoons ground cinnamon, divided

3 tablespoons freshly squeezed lemon juice, divided

1/4 teaspoon ground nutmeg

1 scoop vanilla bone broth protein

2 cups whole shelled walnuts

1 cup pitted Medjool dates

Pinch of sea salt

Preheat the oven to 375°F.

In a food processor, combine 2 apples, the raisins, 1 teaspoon of the cinnamon, 1 tablespoon of the lemon juice, the nutmeg, and the bone broth protein and process until smooth and all ingredients are fully incorporated.

Chop the remaining apples. In a large bowl, toss the chopped apples with the remaining lemon juice. Pour the apple-raisin puree over the apples and mix well.

Spoon the mixture into a 9-inch deep-dish pie plate and set aside.

In the food processor, pulse the walnuts, dates, salt, and remaining cinnamon until coarsely ground.

Sprinkle the mixture over the apples and press down lightly with your hands.

Bake for 30 minutes and serve.

BANANA CHIA PUDDING

SERVINGS: 3–4

TIME: 30 MINUTES

1 cup full-fat unsweetened canned coconut milk

¼ cup ground chia seeds

5 tablespoons raw honey

1 banana

1 scoop vanilla bone broth protein

¼ teaspoon pumpkin pie spice or ground cinnamon

Place all the ingredients in a food processor or blender and process for 1 minute.

Refrigerate for 10–15 minutes before serving.

CACAO BLUEBERRY ICE CREAM

SERVINGS: 8

TIME: 3½ HOURS

1 (15-ounce) can full-fat unsweetened coconut milk

¾ cup water

⅔ cup maple sugar

⅔ cup cacao powder

1 teaspoon vanilla extract

½ teaspoon sea salt

1 pint fresh blueberries

In a small saucepan over medium-high heat, whisk together all the ingredients except the blueberries. Bring to a simmer and whisk until the sugar has dissolved. Remove from the heat.

Pour the mixture into a glass container or mixing bowl and place in the refrigerator. Let it chill for 2–3 hours.

Remove the mixture from the refrigerator and pour into a chilled ice cream maker. Churn for 20 minutes. Add the blueberries and churn for another 5 minutes. Return the mixture to the mixing bowl and freeze for 1 hour.

CARROT CAKE SQUARES

SERVINGS: 10
TIME: 35 MINUTES

1 cup pitted Medjool date halves
½ cup coconut oil, melted
1 teaspoon vanilla extract
2 teaspoons ground cinnamon
2 large eggs
¼ teaspoon sea salt
¾ cup vanilla bone broth protein
1½ cups shredded carrots
½ cup coarsely chopped walnuts
1½ cups rolled oats
¾ cup raisins

Preheat the oven to 375°F.

Line an 8 × 8-inch baking dish with parchment paper.

In a food processor, combine the dates, coconut oil, vanilla, and cinnamon. Process until well combined.

In a medium bowl, whisk together the eggs, salt, and bone broth protein until well combined.

Add the date mixture to the egg mixture and stir until incorporated.

Add the remaining ingredients and mix well.

Transfer to the baking dish and bake for 20–25 minutes, or until golden brown on the outside.

MOCK CHEESECAKE PUDDING

SERVINGS: 2
TIME: 5 MINUTES

1 cup cashew butter
1/3 cup freshly squeezed lemon juice
1/3 cup raw honey
4 pitted Medjool dates
1 teaspoon vanilla extract
1/2 teaspoon sea salt

In a high-powered blender, puree all ingredients until smooth. Serve immediately or chill 2–3 hours before serving.

COCONUT CHIA PUDDING

SERVINGS: 2

TIME: 3¼ HOURS

1 (15-ounce) can full-fat unsweetened coconut milk

¼ cup ground chia seeds

10–12 drops liquid stevia

2 scoops collagen protein (optional)

Sliced kiwifruit, berries, cacao nibs, sliced bananas, or goji
     berries for garnish (optional)

In a small bowl, mix the coconut milk, chia seeds,
stevia, and collagen protein (if using). Let sit at least 2–3
hours in the refrigerator, or as long as overnight, until the
mixture has thickened and achieved a puddinglike
consistency.

Divide the pudding into two bowls. Serve with optional
garnishes or enjoy it plain.

KEY LIME PIE

SERVINGS: 6–8
TIME: 2¼ HOURS

FOR THE CRUST

3 cups raw whole shelled walnuts
2 cups pitted Medjool dates
1 teaspoon vanilla extract
Pinch of sea salt

FOR THE FILLING

1¼ cups raw cashews, soaked in water overnight
1 scoop collagen protein
Zest of 2 limes
¼ teaspoon sea salt
1 cup pitted Medjool dates
1 tablespoon raw honey
1 tablespoon melted coconut oil
2 tablespoons freshly squeezed lime juice

In a food processor, combine the crust ingredients and process until the mixture becomes a dough.

Spread the dough out evenly in the bottom of an ungreased 9-inch springform pan. Place the pan in the freezer for 30 minutes.

In a high-powered blender, blend all the filling ingredients on low speed until well combined.

Remove the crust from the freezer. Pour the filling mixture on top of the crust, cover the pan, and return the pie to the freezer.

Freeze for at least 2 hours. Defrost the pie in the refrigerator for 20 minutes before serving.

NO-BAKE CASHEW TRUFFLES

SERVINGS: 6–8
TIME: 10 MINUTES

1 cup raw cashews
2 tablespoons cashew butter
6 pitted Medjool dates
1½ teaspoons ground cinnamon, divided
1 teaspoon vanilla extract
3 tablespoons coconut oil, melted and cooled
1 tablespoon full-fat unsweetened canned coconut milk
3–4 scoops chocolate bone broth protein

In a food processor, process the cashews until small chunks form. Add the cashew butter, dates, ½ teaspoon cinnamon, vanilla, coconut oil, coconut milk, and bone broth protein, blending until the mixture achieves a pastelike consistency.

Using your hands, roll the dough into 6–8 bite-size balls.

Dust with 1 teaspoon cinnamon and chill in the refrigerator for 1 hour, or until firm.

NO-BAKE CHOCOLATE CHIP COOKIES

SERVINGS: 6
TIME: 2¼ HOURS

1½ cups almond butter
¼ cup raw honey
1 teaspoon vanilla extract
¼ teaspoon sea salt
1 scoop bone broth protein
½ cup stevia-sweetened chocolate chips (at least 80% cacao)

In a medium bowl, stir together the almond butter, honey, vanilla, and salt. Add the bone broth protein and combine thoroughly.

Stir in the chocolate chips and place the mixture in the refrigerator for about 2 hours.

Remove from the refrigerator, form into cookie shapes, and enjoy.

NO-BAKE PUMPKIN PIE

SERVINGS: 6–8
TIME: 10 MINUTES

FOR THE CRUST

2 cups pecan or walnut halves
½ cup pitted Medjool dates, soaked in water for 30 minutes
Pinch of sea salt

FOR THE FILLING

2 cups canned pumpkin puree

1 cup pitted Medjool dates, soaked in water for 30
   minutes

¼ cup unsweetened almond milk or water

2 teaspoons ground cinnamon

1 teaspoon grated fresh ginger

1 teaspoon ground nutmeg

1 teaspoon coconut oil

Dash of vanilla extract

In a food processor, blend the crust ingredients until well combined.

Pat the mixture evenly onto the bottom and sides of a 9-inch pie plate, pressing gently with your fingers.

In a high-powered blender, puree the filling ingredients until thoroughly combined and smooth.

Pour the filling into the crust. Refrigerate for at least 1 hour before serving.

RASPBERRY ICE CREAM

SERVINGS: 4

TIME: 1 HOUR

1¾ cups full-fat unsweetened canned coconut milk

5 pitted Medjool dates, halved

1 scoop collagen protein

½ teaspoon vanilla extract

2½ cups fresh or frozen raspberries

2 tablespoons freshly squeezed lemon juice

¾ teaspoon lemon zest

In a high-powered blender, puree the coconut milk, dates, and collagen protein until completely smooth.

Add the vanilla, raspberries, lemon juice, and lemon zest. Puree on high speed until well blended.

Pour the mixture into a glass container and store in the freezer for an hour. Then transfer the mixture to an ice cream maker and prepare according to the manufacturer's instructions.

Transfer the ice cream to a large glass container with a lid and freeze for at least 1 hour or overnight.

CHAPTER 14

Your Simple, One-Stop Guide to Basic Collagen-Related Info

Answers to the 13 Most Common Questions

Life is busy, and retaining all the information I've given you about collagen can be tricky, so I want to leave you with a quick and simple summary of some of the most important things you need to know. Here are answers to the thirteen questions I get asked most frequently.

WHAT DO THE DIFFERENT TYPES OF COLLAGEN DO FOR YOU?

There are many different types of collagen. The most common are I, II, III, V, and X. Here's a quick overview of each:

■ Type I collagen is the most abundant type found in the human body. It's in your bones, teeth, skin, ligaments, tendons, cartilage, and the disks between vertebrae. By consuming type I collagen, you can promote skin health and normal wound healing, as well as lean muscle mass and digestive health.

■ Type II collagen is provided in the highest concentrations from chicken collagen. It helps form cartilage, safeguards joint health, and supports the organs and the respiratory system.

■ Type III collagen usually occurs with, and supports, type I collagen. It plays an integral role in the health of the intestines, heart, blood vessels, and muscles.

■ Type V collagen helps form tissues of the liver, lungs, muscles, bones, and the placenta in pregnant women. It also supports the structure of trillions of cells.

■ Type X collagen helps promote bone strength and supports cartilage maintenance.

IF MY BODY ALREADY MAKES COLLAGEN, WHY DO I NEED TO CONSUME MORE?

Your levels of collagen-rich tissues wane as you age, and your body begins producing less—a double whammy that leaves you more and more in need of dietary collagen. Collagen production also suffers when you're very active, sick, dealing with a lot of stress, or exposed to other collagen-depleting factors, like an autoimmune illness, excessive sun exposure, poor diet, or smoking—second- or firsthand.

HOW DID OUR ANCESTORS (OR PEOPLE EATING TRADITIONAL DIETS) CONSUME COLLAGEN?

Throughout history, people obtained collagen by consuming real bone broth, and, along with it, nearly every part of the animal. People ate nose to tail, meaning they consumed bone marrow, organ meats, skin, the small bones found in fish, and so on. In contrast, our modern diet includes little collagen, because we consume lots of muscle meat and/or conventional protein supplements but usually discard other valuable animal parts.

WHAT ARE THE BEST SOURCES OF COLLAGEN?

Real bone broth—made with the bones, skin, connective tissue, and organ meats of animals—is my favorite. Other great alternatives are hydrolyzed collagen supplements made from ingredients like beef collagen, chicken collagen, eggshell membrane collagen, and fish collagen. Taking collagen supplements rather than consuming collagen naturally from foods is similar to getting other nutrients, such as vitamins and minerals, from supplements. Real foods contain more than a single nutrient and are more complex. In this case, bone broth, for example, provides not only collagen but also minerals and antioxidants. It's best to try to get nutrients from real food sources whenever possible. However, collagen supplements can come in handy, because they're convenient. They make it simple to increase your collagen intake. Plus, a good-quality collagen supplement will provide multiple types of collagen (such as types I, II, III, V, and X), along with collagen cofactors such as chondroitin and glutamine. If you're using a collagen supplement, it's important to purchase one that's sourced from whole foods.

ARE THERE VEGETARIAN/VEGAN ALTERNATIVES TO COLLAGEN?

Unfortunately, there is no plant-based option that offers all of the benefits of collagen. Collagen is a unique protein found only in animals. That said, vegetarians and vegans can support collagen production by eating collagen-boosting nutrients, such as those listed in Chapter 5. Eating enough protein daily is important to support your internal production of collagen as well. I recommend eating pasture-raised eggs, organic dairy products (raw, if possible), and fish in order to get enough "complete protein" in your diet and also to obtain small amounts of collagen. If you strictly avoid all animal-derived foods, be sure to get plenty of protein each day from different plant sources, such as nuts, seeds, legumes, 100 percent whole/ancient grains, or plant-based protein powder.

WHAT ARE COLLAGEN SUPPLEMENTS MADE FROM?

Collagen is a protein made up of amino acids. It is found throughout the human body as well as the bodies of other animals. To make collagen supplements, manufacturers derive collagen from dried, concentrated real bone broth or animal parts, including bones, skin, organ meats, scales and fins (in the case of fish), and other types of connective tissue. These parts are typically cleaned, soaked to separate fat, and then soaked in an alkaline or acid solution to help release the collagen. The collagen is then evaporated and milled to help form a fine, consistent powder that is easy for the body to absorb and utilize. Collagen is most often sourced from chickens and cattle but can also come from pigs and other animals; from fish, shellfish, and jellyfish; and from eggshells.

DOES COLLAGEN INTERACT WITH ANY MEDICATIONS?

Because it's a natural protein already found in the body, collagen should not interfere with medications. That said, some people need to follow lower-protein diets due to certain health conditions involving the kidneys and liver, as well as genetic conditions that make it harder to digest protein properly. If you have concerns about taking collagen supplements, you should talk to your physician.

IS COLLAGEN SAFE TO CONSUME DURING PREGNANCY OR WHILE BREASTFEEDING?

As with other protein powders, collagen protein is generally considered safe during pregnancy or while breast-feeding. For thousands of years, many traditional cultures around the world have considered collagen-containing foods, like bone broth and animal organs, to be highly nutritious for pregnant women and new mothers. However, it's always best to speak with your physician before starting any new diet or supplement plan.

WHAT MAKES COLLAGEN POWDER DIFFERENT FROM OTHER PROTEIN POWDERS?

Collagen is unique, due to the amino acids it contains. It is especially high in glycine, proline, and arginine, which many other protein powders are missing or contain in minuscule amounts. But like other protein powders, collagen can be a good post-workout option. Glycine, for instance, interacts with glutamine and cysteine to produce an important antioxidant called glutathione. It also helps with the synthesis of creatine, which is important for muscle building, athletic performance, and energy output. Hydrolyzed collagen protein is easy to digest, because the amino acids are already broken down, making it a great option for people who react poorly to other protein powders.

HOW ARE COLLAGEN AND CALCIUM COFACTORS INVOLVED IN MAINTAINING BONE STRENGTH?

Bone is a living, growing tissue that is mostly made of collagen and is constantly being broken down and renewed. Collagen is a protein that supports the bone-building process by encouraging stem cells to turn into bone cells and proliferate. Calcium and other minerals like phosphate add strength to bones and help them to harden. More than 99 percent of the body's calcium is contained in the bones and teeth. The combination of collagen and calcium supports bone strength and integrity.

SHOULD I USE COLLAGEN POWDER AS A MEAL REPLACEMENT?

Collagen powder is a dietary supplement, not a meal replacement. However, you can make a collagen shake or smoothie with a variety of ingredients that will serve as a healthy meal, and bone broth provides the basis of hearty soups and stews that are full-fledged, satisfying meals.

HOW LONG WILL MY COLLAGEN POWDER LAST, AND WHERE SHOULD I STORE IT?

Collagen powder will last several years. Always check the "best by" date on the product you purchase. Store collagen powder at room temperature in a dry location where it's not exposed to direct sunlight.

ARE THERE ANY SIDE EFFECTS ASSOCIATED WITH CONSUMING COLLAGEN SUPPLEMENTS?

Collagen is easy to digest and rarely causes side effects. A minority of people experience mild indigestion as they're getting used to the product. If you feel gassy, bloated, or constipated, cut your collagen in half, then gradually increase your daily servings.

The Collagen Diet for Life

Final Thoughts as You Move Forward

If you're feeling great after your 28-day collagen diet comes to a close, I encourage you to continue following the plan's basic guidelines and using your favorite recipes. Because the program is built around whole foods, juicing, and fasting, as well as healthy sources of collagen, it's an approach you can maintain for life.

If you want to introduce more variety into your diet, you can easily do so and still maintain your weight and bolster collagen by transitioning to a modified plan that includes plenty of the collagen-rich and nutrient-dense foods mentioned throughout this book.

I recommend that you continue to practice intermittent fasting, because it confers such a wide range of health benefits. Choose the approach that fits with your life and feels right to you, whether it's fasting daily (by eating within an eight- or nine-hour window and then fasting for fifteen to sixteen hours) or having a once-weekly cleanse day. In order to refresh your body, you should consider periodic three-day, liquid-only cleanses throughout the year. Chelsea and I do it twice a year. It leaves us feeling energetic, recharged, and able to think more clearly and function at our best.

If you find yourself reverting to old habits that don't serve you, or if you're gaining weight or feeling fatigued, consider simply restarting the 3-day cleanse and repeating the 28-day meal plan. No matter what type of diet you decide to follow for the long term, I urge you to include collagen in your daily repertoire. So long as you continue using it, it will provide benefits for your metabolism, joints, muscles, and skin—tissues that are integral to your health and well-being.

I know you're as concerned about healthy aging as I am. I believe that collagen will give us all the best shot at staying pain-free and active, avoiding the common problems and pitfalls that crop up with age—and achieving lifelong wellness. May we all reach that goal together.

Acknowledgments

Books never come into being without the hard work of lots of people, and this one is no exception. I'm grateful to Ginny Graves, for her superb work helping me craft this book. My sincerest thanks to Bonnie Solow, my literary agent, who always has my back and is the smartest in the business, and to Tracy Behar, editor extraordinaire, and her wonderful team at Little, Brown Spark, for their keen editing, thoughtful guidance, and deep dedication to bringing readers the best nutrition and health information available. I also owe a debt of gratitude to my dear friend and business partner Jordan Rubin, who encouraged me to write this book and served as an ever-present sounding board and source of support—and to my entire team at Ancient Nutrition, whose hard work and enthusiasm are as inspiring as they are gratifying. Finally, to the people who follow me on social media, fans of my website, and readers of this book: You're the reason I've dedicated my life to healing, and you have my heartfelt gratitude.

Big Blessings!
Josh Axe

Notes

1. Hongdong Song, Siqi Zhang, Ling Zhang, Bo Li, "Effect of Orally Administered Collagen Peptides from Bovine Bone on Skin Aging in Chronologically Aged Mice," *Nutrients* 9 (2017).

2. D. Konig, S. Oesser, S. Scharla, et al., "Specific Collagen Peptides Improve Bone Mineral Density and Bone Markers in Postmenopausal Women—A Randomized Controlled Study," *Nutrients* 10 (2018).

3. F. D. Choi, C. T. Sung, M. L. Juhasz, et al., "Oral Collagen Supplementation: A Systematic Review of Dermatological Applications," *Journal of Drugs in Dermatology* 18 (2019): 9–16.

4. Ian J. Wallace, Steven Worthington, David T. Felson, et al., "Knee Osteoarthritis Has Doubled in Prevalence Since the Mid-20th Century," *PNAS Proceedings of the National Academy of Sciences* 114 (2017): 9332–9336.

5. Centers for Disease Control and Prevention, Arthritis National Statistics, February 2018, https://www.cdc.gov/arthritis/data_statistics/national-statistics.html.

6. Stephanie L. Schnorr, Marco Candela, Simone Rampelli, et al., "Gut Microbiome of the Hadza Hunter-Gatherers," *Nature Communications* 5 (2014).

7. Eric P. Plaisance, Frank L. Greenway, Anik Boudreau, et al., "Dietary Methionine Restriction Increases Fat Oxidation in Obese Adults with Metabolic Syndrome," *Journal of Clinical Endocrinology & Metabolism* 96 (2011): E836–E840.

8. J. K. Virtanen, S. Voutilainen, T. H. Rissanen, et al., "High Dietary Methionine Intake Increases the Risk of Acute Coronary Events in

Middle-Aged Men," *Nutrition, Metabolism & Cardiovascular Disease* 16 (2006): 113–120.

9. Wataru Yamadera, Kentaru Inagawa, Shinaro Chiba, et al., "Glycine Ingestion Improves Subjective Sleep Quality in Human Volunteers, Correlating with Polysomnographic Changes," *Sleep and Biological Rhythms* 5 (2007): 126–131.

10. Osamu Hashizume, Sakiko Ohnishi, Takayuki Mito, et al., "Epigenetic Regulation of the Nuclear-Coded GCAT and SHMT2 Genes Confers Human Age-Associated Mitochondrial Respiration Defects," *Scientific Reports* 5 (2015).

11. Yasutaka Shigemura, Daiki Kubomura, Yoshio Sato, et al. "Dose-Dependent Changes in the Levels of Free and Peptide Forms of Hydroxyproline in Human Plasma after Collagen Hydrolysate Ingestion," *Food Chemistry* 159 (2014): 328–332.

12. T. Kawaguchi, P. N. Nanbu, and M. Kurokawa, "Distribution of Prolylhydroxyproline and Its Metabolites after Oral Administration in Rats," *Biological and Pharmaceutical Bulletin* 35 (2012): 422–427.

13. Jerome Asserin, Elian Lati, Toshiaki Shioya, et al., "The Effect of Oral Collagen Peptide Supplementation on Skin Moisture and the Dermal Collagen Network: Evidence from an *Ex Vivo* Model and Randomized, Placebo-Controlled Clinical Trials," *Journal of Cosmetic Dermatology* 14 (2015): 291–301.

14. L. Duteil, C. Queille Roussel, Y. Maubert, et al., "Specific Natural Bioactive Type I Collagen Peptides Oral Intake Reverse Skin Aging Signs in Mature Women," *Journal of Aging Research & Clinical Practice* (2016).

15. A. E. Postlethwaite, W. K. Wong, P. Clements, et al., "A Multicenter, Randomized, Double-Blind, Placebo-Controlled Trial of Oral Type I Collagen Treatment in Patients with Diffuse Cutaneous Systemic Sclerosis: Oral Type I Collagen Does Not Improve Skin in All Patients, but May Improve Skin in Late-Phase Disease," *Arthritis & Rheumatology* 58 (2008): 1810–1822.

16. Q. A. Dar, E. M. Schott, S. E. Catheline, et al., "Daily Oral Con-

sumption of Hydrolyzed Type I Collagen Is Chondroprotective and Anti-inflammatory in Murine Posttraumatic Osteoarthritis," *PLOS One* 12 (2017).

17. David C. Crowley, Francis C. Lau, Prachi Sharma, et al., "Safety and Efficacy of Undenatured Type II Collagen in the Treatment of Osteoarthritis of the Knee: A Clinical Trial," *International Journal of Medical Sciences* 6 (2009): 312–321.

18. David E. Trentham, Roselynn A. Dynesius-Trentham, E. John Orav, et al., "Effects of Oral Administration of Type II Collagen on Rheumatoid Arthritis," *Science* 261 (1993): 1727–1730.

19. P. Betz, A. Nerlich, J. Wilske, et al., "The Time-Dependent Rearrangement of the Epithelial Basement Membrane in Human Skin Wounds — Immunohistochemical Localization of Collagen IV and VII," *International Journal of Legal Medicine* 105 (1992): 93–97.

20. M. M. Hurley, D. J. Adams, L. Wang, et al., "Accelerated Fracture Healing in Transgenic Mice Overexpressing Anabolic Isoform of Fibroblast Growth Factor 2," *Journal of Cell Biochemistry* 117 (2016): 599–611.

21. Daniel O. Clegg, Domenic J. Reda, Crystal L. Harris, et al., "Glucosamine, Chondroitin Sulfate, and the Two in Combination for Painful Knee Osteoarthritis," *New England Journal of Medicine* 354 (2006): 795–808.

22. M. Rizwan, I. Rodriguez-Blanco, A. Harbottle, et al., "Tomato Paste Rich in Lycopene Protects against Cutaneous Photodamage in Humans In Vivo: A Randomized Controlled Trial," *British Journal of Dermatology* 164 (2011): 154–162.

23. J. Orbe, J. A. Rodriguez, R. Arias, et al., "Antioxidant Vitamins Increase the Collagen Content and Reduce MMP-1 in a Porcine Model of Atherosclerosis: Implications for Plaque Stabilization," *Atherosclerosis* 167 (2003): 45–53.

24. L. S. McAnulty, D. C. Nieman, C. L. Dumke, et al., "Effect of Blueberry Ingestion on Natural Killer Cell Counts, Oxidative Stress, and Inflammation Prior to and after 2.5 H of Running," *Applied Physiology, Nutrition and Metabolism* 36 (2011): 976–984.

25. V. E. Reeve, M. Allanson, S. J. Arun, et al., "Mice Drinking Goji Berry Juice (Lycium Barbarum) Are Protected from UV Radiation-Induced Skin Damage via Antioxidant Pathways," *Photochemical & Photobiological Sciences* 9 (2010): 601–607.

26. B. O. Rennard, R. F. Ertl, G. L. Gossman, et al., "Chicken Soup Inhibits Neutrophil Chemotaxis In Vitro," *Chest* 118 (2000): 1150–1157.

27. Bin Shan, Yizhong Z. Cai, Mei Sun, et al., "Antioxidant Capacity of 26 Spice Extracts and Characterization of Their Phenolic Constituents," *Journal of Agricultural and Food Chemistry* 53 (2005): 7749–7759.

28. G. de Almeida Goncalves, A. B. de Sa-Nakanishi, J. F. Comar, et al., "Water Soluble Compounds of Rosmarinus Officinalis L. Improve the Oxidative and Inflammatory States of Rats with Adjuvant-Induced Arthritis," *Food and Function* 25 (2018): 2328–2340.

29. M. A. Khan, M. Subramaneyaan, V. K. Arora, et al., "Effect of Withania Somnifera (Ashwagandha) Root Extract on Amelioration of Oxidative Stress and Autoantibodies Production in Collagen-Induced Arthritic Rats," *Journal of Complementary and Integrative Medicine* 12 (2015): 117–125.

30. A. H. Kwon, Z. Qiu, M. Hashimoto, et al., "Effects of Medicinal Mushroom (Sparassis Crispa) on Wound Healing in Streptozotocin-Induced Diabetic Rats," *American Journal of Surgery* 197 (2009): 503–509.

31. B. H. Marouf, S. A. Hussain, Z. S. Ali, et al., "Resveratrol Supplementation Reduces Pain and Inflammation in Knee Osteoarthritis Patients Treated with Meloxicam: A Randomized Placebo-Controlled Trial," *Journal of Medicinal Food* (2018).

32. Stoyan Dimitrov, Elaine Hulteng, and Suzi Hong, "Inflammation and Exercise: Inhibition of Monocytic TNF Production by Acute Exercise Via B2-Adrenergic Activation," *Brain, Behavior and Immunity* 61 (2017): 60–68.

33. Bente Klarlund Pedersen, "Anti-inflammatory Effects of Exercise: Role in Diabetes and Cardiovascular Disease," *European Journal of Clinical Investigation* 47 (2017): 600–611.

34. S. Y. Xu, Y. B. He, S. Y. Deng, et al., "Intensity-Dependent Effect

of Treadmill Running on Rat Achilles Tendon," *Experimental and Therapeutic Medicine* 15 (2018): 5377–5383.

35. G. X. Ni, S. Y. Liu, L. Lei, et al., "Intensity-Dependent Effect of Treadmill Running on Knee Articular Cartilage in a Rat Model," *BioMed Research International* 2013 (2013).

36. Grant S. Shields, Shari Young Kuchenbacker, Sarah D. Pressman, et al., "Better Cognitive Control of Emotional Information Is Associated with Reduced Pro-inflammatory Cytokine Reactivity to Emotional Stress," *Stress* 19 (2016): 63–68.

37. J. D. Creswell, A. A. Taren, E. K. Lindsay, et al., "Alterations in Resting-State Functional Connectivity Link Mindfulness Meditation with Reduced Interleukin-6: A Randomized Controlled Trial," *Biological Psychiatry* 80 (2016): 53–61.

38. D. S. Black, S. W. Cole, M. R. Irwin, et al., "Yogic Meditation Reverses NF-kB and IRF-Related Transcriptome Dynamics in Leukocytes of Family Dementia Caregivers in a Randomized Controlled Trial," *Psychoneuroimmunology* 38 (2013): 348–355.

39. S. Amin, J. Niu, A. Guermazi, et al., "Cigarette Smoking and the Risk for Cartilage Loss and Knee Pain in Men with Knee Osteoarthritis," *Annals of the Rheumatic Diseases* 66 (2007): 18–22.

40. F. Davatchi, B. S. Abdollahi, M. Mohyeddin, et al., "Mesenchymal Stem Cell Therapy for Knee Osteoarthritis: Preliminary Report in Four Patients," *International Journal of Rheumatic Diseases* 14 (2011): 211–215; F. Davatchi, B. Sadeghi Abdollahi, M. Mohyeddin, et al., "Mesenchymal Stem Cell Therapy for Knee Osteoarthritis: 5 Years Follow-Up of Three Patients," *International Journal of Rheumatic Diseases* 19 (2016): 219–225.

41. A. Vega, M. A. Martin-Ferrero, F. Del Canto, et al., "Treatment of Knee Osteoarthritis with Allogeneic Bone Marrow Mesenchymal Stem Cells: A Randomized Controlled Trial," *Transplantation* 99 (2015): 1681–1690.

42. C. Cramer, E. Freisinger, R. K. Jones, et al., "Persistent High Glucose Concentrations Alter the Regenerative Potential of Mesenchymal Stem Cells," *Stem Cells and Development* 19 (2010): 1875–1884.

43. T. Lo, J. H. Ho, M. H. Yang, et al., "Glucose Reduction Prevents Replicative Senescence and Increases Mitochondrial Respiration in Human Mesenchymal Stem Cells," *Cell Transplantation* 20 (2011): 813–825.

44. M. M. Mihaylova, C. W. Cheng, A. Q. Cao, et al., "Fasting Activates Fatty Acid Oxidation to Enhance Intestinal Stem Cell Function during Homeostatis and Aging," *Cell Stem Cell* 22 (2018): 769–778.

45. Massimiliano Cerletti, Young C. Jang, Lydia W. S. Finley, et al., "Short-Term Calorie Restriction Enhances Skeletal Muscle Stem Cell Function," *Cell Stem Cell* 10 (2012): 515–519.

46. Monika Maredziak, Agnieszka Smieszek, Klaudia Chrzastek, et al., "Physical Activity Increases the Total Number of Bone-Marrow-Derived Mesenchymal Stem Cells, Enhances Their Osteogenic Potential, and Inhibits Their Adipogenic Properties," *Stem Cells International* (2015).

47. Asya Rolls, Wendy W. Pang, Ingrid Ibarra, et al., "Sleep Deprivation Impairs Haematopoietic Stem Cell Transplantation in Mice," *Nature Communications* 6 (2015).

48. X. Yang, Z. P. Han, S. S. Zhan, et al., "Chronic Restraint Stress Decreases the Repair Potential from Mesenchymal Stem Cells on Liver Injury by Inhibiting TGF-B1 Generation," *Cell Death Discovery* 5 (2014).

49. S. Hsu, W. B. Bollag, J. Lewis, et al., "Green Tea Polyphenols Induce Differentiation and Proliferation in Epidermal Keratinocytes," *Journal of Pharmacology and Experimental Therapeutics* 306 (2003): 29–34.

50. Adam D. Bachstetter, Jennifer Jemberg, Andrea Schlunk, et al., "Spirulina Promotes Stem Cell Genesis and Protects against LPS Induced Declines in Neural Stem Cell Proliferation," *PLOS One* 5 (2010).

51. Lei Zhu, Ya-Jun Liu, Hong Shen, et al., "Astragalus and Baicalein Regulate Inflammation of Mesenchymal Stem Cells by the Mitogen-Activated Protein Kinase (MAPK)/ERK Pathway," *Medical Science Monitor* 23 (2017): 3209–3216.

52. Q. Li, W. Xing, X. Gong, et al., "Astragalus Polysaccharide Promotes Proliferation and Osteogenic Differentiation of Bone Mesenchymal Stem Cells by Down-Regulation of MicroRNA-152," *Biomedicine & Pharmacotherapy* 115 (2019).

53. X. H. Wang, H. W. Du, X. H. Guo, et al., "Rehmannia Glutinosa Oligosaccharide Induces Differentiation of Bone Marrow Mesenchymal Stem Cells into Cardiomyocyte-Like Cells," *Genetic and Molecular Research* 15 (2016).

54. Y. Zhang, Y. Wang, L. Wang, et al., "Effects of Rehmannia Glutinosa Oligosaccharide on Human Adipose-Derived Mesenchymal Stem Cells In Vitro," *Life Sciences* 91 (2012): 1323–1327.

55. E. Proksch, M. Schunk, V. Zague, et al., "Oral Intake of Specific Bioactive Collagen Peptides Reduces Skin Wrinkles and Increases Dermal Matrix Synthesis," *Skin Pharmacology and Physiology* 27 (2014): 113–119.

56. Do-Un Kim, Hee-Chul Chung, Jia Choi, et al., "Oral Intake of Low-Molecular Weight Collagen Peptide Improves Hydration, Elasticity, and Wrinkling in Human Skin: A Randomized, Double-Blind, Placebo-Controlled Study," *Nutrients* 10 (2018).

57. N. Inoue, F. Sugihara, and X. Wang, "Ingestion of Bioactive Collagen Hydrolysates Enhance Facial Skin Moisture and Elasticity and Reduce Facial Aging Signs in a Randomised Double-Blind Placebo-Controlled Clinical Study," *Journal of the Science of Food and Agriculture* 96 (2016): 4077–4081.

58. A. Czajka, E. M. Kania, L. Genovese, et al., "Daily Oral Supplementation with Collagen Peptides Combined with Vitamins and Other Bioactive Compounds Improves Skin Elasticity and Has a Beneficial Effect on Joint and General Wellbeing," *Nutrition Research* 57 (2018): 97–108.

59. Michael Schunck, Vivian Zague, Steffen Oesser, et al., "Dietary Supplementation with Specific Collagen Peptides Has a Body Mass Index-Dependent Beneficial Effect on Cellulite Morphology," *Journal of Medicinal Food* 19 (2015): 1340–1348.

60. Naoki Ito, Shinobu Seki, and Fumitaka Ueda, "Effects of Composite

Supplement Containing Collagen Peptide and Ornithine on Skin Conditions and Plasma IGF-1 Levels—A Randomized, Double-Blind, Placebo-Controlled Trial," *Marine Drugs* 16 (2018).

61. H. Matsumura et al., "Hair Follicle Aging Is Driven by Transepidermal Elimination of Stem Cells via COL17A1 Proteolysis," *Science* 35 (2016).

62. G. Ablon and S. Kogan, "A Six-Month Randomized, Double-Blind, Placebo-Controlled Study Evaluating the Safety and Efficacy of a Nutraceutical Supplement for Promoting Hair Growth in Women with Self-Perceived Thinning Hair," *Journal of Drugs in Dermatology* 17 (2018): 558–565.

63. D. Hexsel et al., "Oral Supplementation with Specific Bioactive Collagen Peptides Improves Nail Growth and Reduces Symptoms of Brittle Nails," *Journal of Cosmetic Dermatology* 16 (2017): 520–526.

64. Alexander Wunsch and Karsten Matuschka, "A Controlled Trial to Determine the Efficacy of Red and Near-Infrared Light Treatment in Patient Satisfaction, Reduction of Fine Lines, Wrinkles, Skin Roughness, and Intradermal Collagen Density Increase," *Photomedicine and Laser Surgery* 32 (2014): 93–100.

65. Pinar Avci, Guarav K. Gupta, Jason Clark, et al., "Low-Level Laser (Light) Therapy (LLLT) for Treatment of Hair Loss," *Lasers in Surgery and Medicine* 46 (2014): 144–151.

66. Matthias C. Aust, Des Fernandes, Perkles Kolokythas, et al., "Percutaneous Collagen Induction Therapy: An Alternative Treatment for Scars, Wrinkles, and Skin Laxity," *Plastic and Reconstructive Surgery* 121 (2008): 1421–1429.

67. Imran Majid, "Microneedling Therapy in Atrophic Facial Scars: An Objective Assessment," *Journal of Cutaneous and Aesthetic Surgery* 2 (2009) 26–30.

68. Rachita Dhurat, M. S. Sukesh, Ganesh Avhad, et al., "A Randomized Evaluator Blinded Study of Effect of Microneedling in Androgenetic Alopecia: A Pilot Study," *International Journal of Trichology* 5 (2013): 6–11.

69. Maha Sellami, Wissem Dhahbi, Lawrence D. Hayes, et al., "Combined Sprint and Resistance Training Abrogates Age Differences in Somatic Hormones," *PLOS One* 12 (2017).

70. S. A. Lim and K. J. Cheong, "Regular Yoga Practice Improves Antioxidant Status, Immune Function and Stress Hormone Releases in Young Healthy People: A Randomized, Double-Blind, Controlled Pilot Study," *Journal of Alternative and Complementary Medicine* 21 (2015): 530–538.

71. Martina Barchitta, Andrea Maugeri, Giuliana Favara, et al., "Nutrition and Wound Healing: An Overview Focusing on the Beneficial Effects of Curcumin," *International Journal of Molecular Sciences* 20 (2019).

72. N. Takasao, K. Tsuji-Naito, S. Ishikura, et al., "Cinnamon Extract Promotes Type I Collagen Biosynthesis via Activition of IGF-I Signaling in Human Dermal Fibroblasts," *Journal of Agricultural and Food Chemistry* 60 (2012): 1193–1200.

73. Narasimharao Bhagavathula, Roscoe L. Warner, Marissa DaSilva, et al., "A Combination of Curcumin and Ginger Extract Improves Abrasion Wound Healing in Corticosteroid-Damaged Hairless Rat Skin," *Wound Repair and Regeneration* 17 (2009).

74. T. Fujii, M. Wakaizumi, T. Ikami, et al., "Amla (*Emblica* Officinalis Gaertn.) Extract Promotes Procollagen Production and Inhibits Matrix Metalloproteinase-1 in Human Skin Fibroblasts," *Journal of Ethnopharmacology* 119 (2008): 53–57.

75. Jongsung Lee, Eunsun Jung, Jiyoung Lee, et al., "Panax Ginseng Induces Human Type I Collagen Synthesis during Activation of Smad Signaling," *Journal of Ethnopharmacology* 109 (2007): 29–34.

76. M. F. Hsu and B. H. Chiang, "Stimulating Effects of Bacillus Subtilis Natto-Fermented Radix Astragali on Hyaluronic Acid Production in Human Skin Cells," *Journal of Ethnopharmacology* 125 (2009): 474–481.

77. Piergiacomo Calzavara-Pinton, Cristina Zane, Elena Facchinetti, et al., "Topical Besellic Acids for Treatment of Photo-Aged Skin," *Dermatologic Therapy* 23 (2010).

78. H. M. Park, E. Moon, M. H. Kim, et al., "Extract of Punica Granatum Inhibits Skin Photoaging Induced by UVB Irradiation," *International Journal of Dermatology* 83 (2007): 276–282.

79. E. Ranato, S. Martinotti, and B. Burlando, "Wound Healing Properties of Jojoba Liquid Wax: An In Vitro Study," *Journal of Ethnopharmacology* 134 (2011): 443–449.

80. Anita Berman, "Looking beyond Gluten Free: Choose a Gut-Supportive Diet for Long-Term Health with Celiac Disease," Gluten Intolerance Group, Winter 2015, https://gluten.org/looking-beyond-gluten-free -choose-gut-supportive-diet-long-term-health-celiac-disease.

81. Alessio Fasano, "Leaky Gut and Autoimmune Disease," *Clinical Reviews in Allergy and Immunology* 42 (2012): 71–78.

82. Ibid.

83. Q. Mu, H. Zhang, and X. M. Luo, "SLE: Another Autoimmune Disorder Influenced by Microbes and Diet?" *Frontiers in Immunology* 6 (2006).

84. Aaron Lerner, Patricia Jeremias, and Thorsten Matthias, "Gut-Thyroid Axis and Celiac Disease," *Endocrine Connections* 6 (2017): R52–R58.

85. Melinda Wenner Moyer, "Gut Bacteria May Play a Role in Autism," *Scientific American,* September 2014, https://www.scientificameri can.com/article/gut-bacteria-may-play-a-role-in-autism/?redirect=1.

86. M. Yamamoto, M. I. Pinto-Sanchez, P. Bercik, et al., "Metabolomics Reveals Elevated Urinary Excretion of Collagen Degradation and Epithelial Cell Turnover Products in Irritable Bowel Syndrome Patients," *Metabolomics* 15 (2019).

87. Yulan Liu, Xiuying Wang, and Chien-An Andy Hu, "Therapeutic Potential of Amino Acids in Inflammatory Bowel Disease," *Nutrients* 9 (2017).

88. Ibid.

89. Ibid.

90. Qianru Chen, Oliver Chen, Isabela M. Martins, et al., "Collagen Peptides Ameliorate Intestinal Epithelial Barrier Dysfunction in

Immunostimulatory Caco-2 Cell Monolayers via Enhancing Tight Junctions," *Food & Function* 3 (2017).

91. Xiao Xu, Xiuying Wang, Huanting Wu, et al., "Glycine Relieves Intestinal Injury by Maintaining mTOR Signaling and Suppressing AMPK, TLR4, and NOD Signaling in Weaned Piglets after Lipopolysaccharide Challenge," *International Journal of Molecular Sciences* 19 (2018).

92. I. Tsune, K. Ikejima, M. Hirose, et al., "Dietary Glycine Prevents Chemical-Induced Experimental Colitis in the Rat," *Gastroenterology* 125 (2003): 775–785.

93. Zhi Zhong, Michael D. Wheeler, Xiangli Li, et al., "L-Glycine: A Novel Antiinflammatory, Immunomodulatory, and Cytoprotective Agent," *Current Opinion in Clinical Nutrition and Metabolic Care* 6 (2003): 229–240.

94. Y. Ji, Z. Dai, S. Sun, et al., "Hyrdoxyproline Attenuates Dextran Sulfate Sodium-Induced Colitis in Mice: Involvement of the NF-kB Signaling and Oxidative Stress," *Molecular Nutrition and Food Research* 62 (2018).

95. J. Bertrand, I. Ghouzali, C. Guerin, et al., "Glutamine Restores Tight Junction Protein Claudin-1 Expression in Colonic Mucosa of Patients with Diarrhea-Predominant Irritable Bowel Syndrome," *Journal of Parenteral and Enteral Nutrition* 40 (2016): 1170–1176.

96. Shanshan Kong, Yanhui H. Zhang, Weiqiang Zhang, et al., "Regulation of Intestinal Epithelial Cells Properties and Functions by Amino Acids," *BioMed Research International* 2018 (2018).

97. Ibid.

98. M. Tariq and A. R. Al Moutaery, "Studies on the Antisecretory, Gastric Anti-Ulcer and Cytoprotective Properties of Glycine," *Research Communications in Molecular Pathology and Pharmacology* 97 (1997): 185–198.

99. G. Sigthorsson, J. Tribble, J. Hayllar, et al., "Intestinal Permeability and Inflammation in Patients on NSAIDs," *Gut* 43 (1989): 506–511.

100. Centers for Disease Control and Prevention, "Joint Pain and Arthritis," September 2018, https://www.cdc.gov/arthritis/pain/index.htm.

101. Centers for Disease Control and Prevention, "Arthritis National Statistics," February 2018, https://www.cdc.gov/arthritis/data_statistics/national-statistics.html.

102. David E. Trentham, Roselynn Dynesius Trentham, E. John Orav, et al., "Effects of Oral Administration of Type II Collagen on Rheumatoid Arthritis," *Science* 261 (1993): 1727–1730.

103. Kenji Sato, "How Collagen Hydrolysate Works on Your Skin and Joints," *Inform* 29 (2018).

104. Ibid.

105. Ibid.

106. O. Bruyere, B. Zegels, L. Leonori, et al., "Effect of Collagen Hydrolysate in Articular Pain: A 6-Month Randomized, Double-Blind, Placebo Controlled Study," *Complementary Therapies in Medicine* 20 (2012): 124–130.

107. P. Benito-Ruiz, M. M. Camacho-Zambrano, J. N. Carrillo-Arcentales, et al., "A Randomized Controlled Trial on the Efficacy and Safety of a Food Ingredient, Collagen Hydrolysate, for Improving Joint Discomfort," *International Journal of Food Sciences and Nutrition* 60 (2009): 99–113.

108. A. Czajka, E. M. Kania, L. Genovese, et al., "Daily Oral Supplementation with Collagen Peptides Combined with Vitamins and Other Bioactive Compounds Improves Skin Elasticity and Has a Beneficial Effect on Joint and General Wellbeing," *Nutrition Research* 57 (2018): 97–108.

109. J. M. Garcia-Coronado, L. Martinez-Olivera, R. E. Elizondo-Omana, et al., "Effect of Collagen Supplementation on Osteoarthritis Symptoms: A Meta-Analysis of Randomized Placebo-Controlled Trials," *International Orthopaedics* 43 (2019): 531–538.

110. Qurratul-Ain Dar, Eric M. Schott, Sarah E. Catherine, et al., "Daily Oral Consumption of Hydrolyzed Type I Collagen Is Chondroprotective and Anti-inflammatory in Murine Posttraumatic Osteoarthritis," *PLOS One* 12 (2017).

111. W. Wei, L. L. Zhang, J. H. Xu, et al., "A Multicenter, Double-Blind, Randomized, Controlled Phase III Clinical Trial of Chicken Type II Collagen in Rheumatoid Arthritis," *Arthritis Research & Therapy* 11 (2009).

112. Ronald J. Maughan, Louise M. Burke, Jiri Dvorak, et al., "IOC Consensus Statement: Dietary Supplements and the High-Performance Athlete," *International Journal of Sport Nutrition and Exercise Metabolism* 28 (2018): 104–125.

113. Kristine L. Clark, Wayne Sebastianelli, Klaus R. Flechsenhar, et al., "24 Week Study on the Use of Collagen Hydrolysate as a Dietary Supplement in Athletes with Activity-Related Joint Pain," *Current Medical Research and Opinion* 24 (2008): 1485–1496.

114. Ibid.

115. Stephan F. E. Praet, Craig R. Purdam, Marijke Welvaert, et al., "Oral Supplementation of Specific Collagen Peptides Combined with Calf-Strengthening Exercises Enhances Function and Reduces Pain in Achilles Tendinopathy Patients," *Nutrients* 11 (2019).

116. Gregory Shaw, Ann Lee-Barthel, Megan L. R. Ross, et al., "Vitamin C–Enriched Gelatin Supplementation before Intermittent Activity Augments Collagen Synthesis," *American Journal of Clinical Nutrition* 105 (2017): 136–143.

117. Linda Rath, "CBD Oil: Should You Try It for Arthritis Symptoms?" Arthritis Foundation, https://www.arthritis.org/living-with-arthritis/treatments/natural/supplements-herbs/cannabidiol-oil.php.

118. Ibid.

119. Ibid.

120. "One in Four Americans Develop Insomnia Each Year," June 8, 2018, https://penntoday.upenn.edu/news/one-four-americans-develops-insomnia-each-year.

121. Wataru Yamadera, Kentaru Inagawa, Shinaro Chiba, et al., "Glycine Ingestion Improves Subjective Sleep Quality in Human Volunteers, Correlating with Polysomnographic Changes," *Sleep and Biological Rhythms* 5 (2007): 126–131.

122. Kentara Inagawa, Takenori Hiraoka, Tohru Kohda, et al., "Subjective Effects of Glycine Ingestion before Bedtime on Sleep Quality," *Sleep and Biological Rhythms* 4 (2006): 75–77.

123. Makoto Bannai and Nobuhiro Kawai, "New Therapeutic Strategy for Amino Acid Medicine: Glycine Improves the Quality of Sleep," *Journal of Pharmacological Sciences* 118 (2012): 145–148.

124. "Facts & Statistics," Anxiety and Depression Association of America, https://adaa.org/about-adaa/press-room/facts-statistics.

125. Makato Bannai, Nobuhiro Kawai, Kenji Nagao, et al., "Oral Administration of Glycine Increases Extracellular Serotonin but Not Dopamine in the Prefrontal Cortex of Rats," *Psychiatry and Clinical Neurosciences* 65 (2011): 142–149.

126. Mareia Valles-Colomer, Gwen Falony, Youssef Darzi, et al., "The Neuroactive Potential of the Human Gut Microbiota in Quality of Life and Depression," *Nature Microbiology* 4 (2019): 623–632.

127. I. G. S. Rubio, G. Castro, A. C. Zanini, et al., "Oral Ingestion of a Hydrolyzed Gelatin Meal in Subjects with Normal Weight and in Obese Patients: Postprandial Effect on Circulating Gut Peptides, Glucose and Insulin," *Eating and Weight Disorders—Studies on Anorexia, Bulimia and Obesity* 13 (2008): 48–53.

128. Mohammed El Hafidi, Israel Perez, Jose Zamora, et al., "Glycine Intake Decreases Plasma Free Fatty Acids, Adipose Cell Size, and Blood Pressure in Sucrose-Fed Rats," *American Journal of Physiology—Regulatory, Integrative and Comparative Physiology* 287 (2004): R1387–R1393.

129. M. K. Caldow et al., "Glycine Supplementation during Calorie Restriction Accelerates Fat Loss and Protects against Further Muscle Loss in Obese Mice," *Clinical Nutrition* 35 (2016): 1118–1126.

130. Ronald J. Maughan, Louise M. Burke, Jiri Dvorak, et al., "IOC Consensus Statement: Dietary Supplements and the High-Performance Athlete," *British Journal of Sports Medicine* 52 (2018): 439–455.

131. Denise Zdzieblik, Steffen Oesser, Manfred W. Baumstark, et al., "Collagen Peptide Supplementation in Combination with Resis-

tance Training Improves Body Composition and Increases Muscle Strength in Elderly Sarcopenic Men: A Randomised Controlled Trial," *British Journal of Nutrition* 114 (2015): 1237–1245.

132. C. P. Earnest, P. G. Snell, R. Rodriguez, et al., "The Effect of Creatine Monohydrate Ingestion on Anaerobic Power Indices, Muscular Strength and Body Composition," *Acta Physiologica Scandinavica* 153 (1995): 207–209.

133. R. H. Boger, S. M. Bode-Boger, W. Thiele, et al., "Restoring Vascular Nitric Oxide Formation by L-Arginine Improves the Symptoms of Intermittent Claudication in Patients with Peripheral Arterial Occlusive Disease," *Journal of the American College of Cardiology* 32 (1995): 1336–1344.

134. T. Tran, D. Bliuc, L. Hansen, et al., "Persistence of Excess Mortality Following Individual Nonhip Fractures: A Relative Survival Analysis," *Journal of Clinical Endocrinology & Metabolism* 103 (2018): 3205–3214.

135. J. M. Beasley, A. Z. LaCroix, J. C. Larson, et al., "Biomarker-Calibrated Protein Intake and Bone Health in the Women's Health Initiative Clinical Trials and Observational Studies," *American Journal of Clinical Nutrition* 99 (2014): 934–940.

136. Daniel Konig, Steffen Oesser, Stephan Scharla, et al., "Specific Collagen Peptides Improve Bone Mineral Density and Bone Markers in Postmenopausal Women—A Randomized Controlled Study," *Nutrients* 10 (2018): 1–11.

137. A. Jennings, A. MacGregor, T. Spector, et al., "Amino Acid Intakes Are Associated with Bone Mineral Density and Prevalence of Low Bone Mass in Women: Evidence from Discordant Monozygotic Twins," *Journal of Bone Mineral Research* 31 (2016): 326–335.

138. American Heart Association and American Stroke Association, "Heart Disease and Stroke Statistics 2018 At-a-Glance," January 2018, https://healthmetrics.heart.org/wp-content/uploads/2018/02/At-A-Glance-Heart-Disease-and-Stroke-Statistics-2018.pdf.

139. Yunpeng Ding, Gard F. T. Swingen, Eva R. Pedersen, et al., "Plasma

Glycine and Risk of Acute Myocardial Infarction in Patients with Suspected Stable Angina Pectoris," *Journal of the American Heart Association* 5 (2015): 1–9.

140. M. El Hafidi, I. Perez, J. Zamora, et al., "Glycine Intake Decreases Plasma Free Fatty Acids, Adipose Cell Size, and Blood Pressure in Sucrose-Fed Rats," *American Journal of Physiology—Regulatory, Integrative and Comparative Physiology* 6 (2004): R1387–R1393.

141. C. Y. Chen, L. C. Ching, Y. J. Liao, et al., "Deficiency of Glycine N-Methyltransferase Aggravates Atherosclerosis in Apolipoprotein E-Null Mice," *Molecular Medicine* 18 (2012): 744–752.

142. M. Adeva-Andany, G. Souto-Adeva, E. Ameneiros-Rodriguez, et al., "Insulin Resistance and Glycine Metabolism in Humans," *Amino Acids* 50 (2018): 11–27.

143. Marc P. McRae, "Therapeutic Benefits of L-Arginine: An Umbrella Review of Meta-Analyses," *Journal of Chiropractic Medicine* 15 (2016): 184–189.

144. Ee-Hwa Kim, Yong-Min Kim, and Jung-Ho Suh, "Effect of Type II Collagen Extract on Immunosuppression Induced by Methotrexate in Rats," *Journal of Exercise Rehabilitation* 14 (2018): 731–738.

145. Roger Geiger, Jan C. Rieckmann, Tobias Wolf, et al., "L-Arginine Modulates T Cell Metabolism and Enhances Survival and Anti-Tumor Activity," *Cell* 167 (2016): 829–842.

146. Karin Schlawicke Engstrom, Ulf Stromberg, Thomas Lundh, et al., "Genetic Variation in Glutathione-Related Genes and Body Burden of Methylmercury," *Environmental Health Perspectives* 116 (2008): 734–739.

147. R. V. Sekhar, S. G. Patel, A. P. Guthikonda, et al., "Deficient Synthesis of Glutathione Underlies Oxidative Stress in Aging and Can Be Corrected by Dietary Cysteine and Glycine Supplementation," *American Journal of Clinical Nutrition* 94 (2011): 847–853.

148. H. A. Feldman, I. Goldstein, D. G. Hatzichristou, et al., "Impotence and Its Medical and Psychological Correlates: Results of the

Massachusetts Male Aging Study," *Journal of Urology* 151 (1994): 54–61.

149. R. Stanislavov and V. Nikolova, "Treatment of Erectile Dysfunction with Pycnogenol and L-Arginine," *Journal of Sex & Marital Therapy* 29 (2003): 207–213.

150. L. M. Westphal, M. L. Polan, A. S. Trant, et al., "A Nutritional Supplement for Improving Fertility in Women: A Pilot Study," *Journal of Reproductive Medicine* 49 (2004): 289–293.

151. Richard A. Miller, David E. Harrison, C. Michael Astle, et al., "Glycine Supplementation Extends Lifespan of Male and Female Mice," *Aging Cell* 18 (2019).

152. Laura M. Perez, Babak Hooshmand, Francesca Mangialesche, et al., "Glutathione Serum Levels and Rate of Multimorbidity Development in Older Adults," *Journals of Gerontology: Biological Sciences* (2019).

153. R. V. Sekhar, S. G. Patel, A. P. Guthikonda, et al., "Deficient Synthesis of Glutathione Underlies Oxidative Stress in Aging and Can Be Corrected by Dietary Cysteine and Glycine Supplementation," *American Journal of Clinical Nutrition* 94 (2011): 847–853.

154. Stephen D. Anton, K. Moehl, W. T. Donahoo, et al., "Flipping the Metabolic Switch: Understanding and Applying Health Benefits of Fasting," *Obesity* 26 (2018): 254–268.

155. Martin P. Wegman, Michael H. Guo, Douglas M. Bennion, et al., "Practicality of Intermittent Fasting in Humans and Its Effects on Oxidative Stress and Genes Related to Aging and Metabolism," *Rejuvenation Research* 18 (2014): 162–172.

156. Kevin D. Hall, Alexis Ayuketah, Robert Brychta, et al., "Ultra-Processed Diets Cause Excess Calorie Intake and Weight Gain: An Inpatient Randomized Controlled Trial of *Ad Libitum* Food Intake," *Cell Metabolism* 30 (2019): 1–11.

About the Author

Dr. Josh Axe, DNM, DC, CNS, is the founder of the world's #1 most visited natural-health website, DrAxe.com. He is also the bestselling author of *Eat Dirt, Keto Diet,* and *Keto Diet Cookbook* and the cofounder of Ancient Nutrition supplement company. Dr. Axe appears regularly on *The Dr. Oz Show* and has written for *Shape, PopSugar, HuffPost, Men's Health, Forbes, Business Insider, Muscle & Fitness Hers,* and *Well+Good.*